Tomography and Cross Sections of the Ear

Tomography and Cross Sections of the Ear

by Galdino E. Valvassori, M. D.
and
Richard A. Buckingham, M. D.

510 partly colored illustrations

1975
W. B. Saunders Company
Philadelphia · London · Toronto

Georg Thieme Publishers
Stuttgart

GALDINO E. VALVASSORI, M.D.

Professor of Radiology,
Abraham Lincoln School of Medicine,
University of Illinois,
Chicago, Ill.

RICHARD A. BUCKINGHAM, M.D.

Clinical Professor of Otolaryngology,
Abraham Lincoln School of Medicine,
University of Illinois,
Chicago, Ill.
Otologist, Resurrection Hospital,
Chicago, Ill.

© 1975 Georg Thieme Verlag, D-7000 Stuttgart 1, Herdweg 63, P. B. 732
Printed in Germany by H. Laupp jr, Tübingen

Library of Congress Catalog Card. Number 74 9443
ISBN 0 7216 8953 1

Dedication

To Sandra

from Galdino, Richard and Mary Grace

Preface

This is an atlas of cross sectional anatomy and pathology of the human temporal bone studied by tomographs, tissue macrosections, and microradiographs.

It is our hope that this work will enable the reader radiologist, otolaryngologist, or anyone interested in the ear to have a better understanding of the temporal bone.

The otologist, using the operating microscope, has learned topographic anatomy of the temporal bone by dissections in the surgical routes.

The radiologist, working with thin body section radiography, has learned to recognize and to appreciate the wealth of fine details demonstrated in the tomographic sections.

In this atlas the otologist will recognize familiar surgical landmarks and can then identify them in the corresponding radiographs.

The radiologist will begin his study with the radiographs and can then recognize structures in the corresponding anatomical macrosections.

Our method of study consists of making tomographs of cadaver temporal bones in one of the six commonly used planes of sectioning. The bones are decalcified and cut into two mm thick macrosections with a commercial meat slicer*. The macrosections are x-rayed with a low intensity machine. The tomographs, photographs of the macrosections, and the microradiographs are studied and compared in order to identify anatomical structures and relationships.

In the comparison of the tomographic sections with photographs of the macrosections, the microradiographs are a natural link and guide between the tomographs and the macrosections.

There are many minute and intricate structures in the small but anatomically complex temporal bone. Tomography is of great clinical value in visualizing the details of the intricate anatomy and complex pathology of the ear. Macrosections and microradiographs enable us to comprehend better the appearance of the normal and abnormal anatomy exposed by the tomographs.

The tomographs were made with the Philips Polytome at the office of Dr. Valvassori. The wet and unmounted macrosections were photographed with Kodachrome film in the laboratory of Dr. Buckingham.

The following persons and organizations have assisted us in the preparation of this Atlas, and we wish to thank them for their valuable help.

From the Department of Otolaryngology of the Abraham Lincoln School of Medicine, University of Illinois, and the Illinois Eye and Ear Infirmary:

Professor Albert H. Andrews, Jr., Head of the Department, who allowed us to use the department facilities; Professor Emeritus Francis L. Lederer, former Head of the Department, who encouraged us; Miss Fannie Lee Billups, who decalcified all of the bones and who did the histology; Mr. Samuel J. Martin, chief medical x-ray technician at the Eye and Ear Infirmary, who made the preliminary drawings of the anatomical sections; Mrs. Helen Facto and Mr. Philip Kott of the Audiovisual Department who assisted with supplemental photography; Dr. Samuel Pruzansky, Professor of Dentistry, who supplied us with some specimens of temporal bones. We are indebted to Professors Edmund A. Petrus and Gleb A. Nedzel, Stritch School of Medicine, Pathologists at Resurrection Hospital, Chicago, Illinois, for anatomical material; Dr. José L. Ferrer, Consulting Otolaryngologist, Resurrection Hospital, Chicago, Illinois, who assisted in the preparation of the specimens.

* U.S. Slicing Machine

From the offices of the authors:
Mrs. William Sullivan and Miss Barbara Buckingham, who provided secretarial help;
Miss Carol J. Klehm, who assisted with radiography.
The final drawings, as they appear in the atlas, are the work of Herr Rudolf Brammer, medical artist of Denzlingen, Germany.
We thank N.V. Philips Gloeilampenfabrieken, Medical Systems Division, Eindhoven, The Netherlands and Philips Medical Systems Inc., Shelton, Connecticut, U.S.A., for the award of a grant to publish the macrosections in color.

We extend our sincere gratitude to Dr. Günther Hauff of the Georg Thieme Verlag for undertaking the publication of our work, and to his colleagues, Herr Achim Menge and Herr Gert Krüger, who assisted in the preparation of this Atlas.

GALDINO E. VALVASSORI, M.D.
RICHARD A. BUCKINGHAM, M.D.

Table of Contents

Techniques

Chapter 1 Tomography, Macrosections, Microsections, and Projections

Tomography of the Temporal Bone

A conventional radiograph is a composite on a single plane of a tri-dimensional structure or body. Each point on the x-ray film shows the summation of all points crossed by the incident x-ray beam as it travels through the body under examination.

In conventional radiography of the temporal bone, small structures are lost in the confusing superimposition of larger structures, and dense or more calcified structures will obscure those of lesser density. Superimposition of some structures may be avoided by predetermined angulation of the head or of the x-ray beam as is done with special projections such as the Schüller, Owen and Chausse. However, some special projections, while improving visualization of certain ear structures, cause disturbing geometrical distortion of the overall appearance of the temporal bone.

The introduction of body section radiography in the late 30's appeared to offer a solution to the problem of radiographic delineation of the extremely small structures of the ear. But a practical application to the study of the temporal bone did not come until over 20 years later with refinement of the radiographic equipment. Body section radiography or tomography is a system in which the x-ray focus and the film move in opposite directions with a constant ratio between their velocities. The film describes a translational motion in relation to the object. In such a system, the x-rays incident on a fixed point on the film have a point of intersection which remains stationary in relation to the object during the exposure. As each point on the film has a point of intersection, all points of intersection will form a plane, the focal plane.

The thickness of each section is inversely proportional to the angle of the scanning movement. The cancellation of the structures outside of the focal plane depends upon the shape and the length of the trajectory of the x-ray source and the film.

Unidirectional or linear body section radiography fails to produce acceptable results in the temporal bone where the structures being investigated are too minute and too close together. The disadvantage of linear tomography is that the effacement of the structures outside of the focal plane is totally uneven. The effacement varies from total effacement of structures whose long axis is perpendicular to the direction of the trajectory to no effacement of structures parallel to the direction of the trajectory.

The study of new patterns of motion led to the construction of new equipment with multi-directional trajectories. At first, circular and elliptical patterns became available. To further improve the coefficient of effacement by increasing the length of the trajectory, more complicated patterns were devised, such as the hypocycloidal and spiral.

Several multi-directional tomographic units are now commercially available. In our study we employed the Philips Polytome which follows a clover-leaf or hypocycloidal trajectory. The 48° angle of the scanning movement produces a focal plane of about 1 mm in thickness. The distance from the focal plane to the film is 35 centimeters, which accounts for a constant 30 % magnification of the objects. For this reason, a small focal spot, 0.3 or 0.6 mm, should be used.

In this study, multiple sections were obtained through isolated temporal bones, 1 mm apart, in one of the six selected projections. The factors employed were the following: 10 Ma, 6 seconds, 48 to 55 Kv with the addition of a 1 mm aluminium and 0.3 mm copper filter. Nine sections were obtained on each 10 × 12 inch film, using a small port size which measured 5 × 5 cm on the film. A combination of Philips par speed screens and Kodak Blue Brand films were employed. Each film was processed in a Kodak automatic processor with a 7 minute cycle.

Macrosections of the Human Temporal Bone

We have found 2 mm thick decalcified sections extremely useful in understanding the anatomy and structural relationships of the intricate and complex human temporal bone.

By obtaining tomographs of the temporal bone before decalcification, and by making microradiographs of the 2 mm thick tissue sections after decalcification and sectioning, we were able to correlate radiographic and anatomic findings accurately and precisely.

Sections 2 mm thick are not histological sections, but rather macrosections. The Zeiss operating microscope and the projection of Kodachrome transparencies of the sections permit examination at magnifications up to 25 times of the unstained macrosections. At these magnifications we can visualize almost all of the macro-anatomy of the temporal bone, although we cannot visualize such histologic features as the organ of Corti or the cellular details of the macula of the utricle and saccule.

The usual 15–25 μ histologic sections of the temporal bone are so thin that they do not give a sense of the spatial relationships of the structures of the ear.

Technique

For this study we removed temporal bones from cadavers at post mortem by using four straight saw cuts. The lateral and medial cuts were parallel to the sagittal plane. These sagittal saw cuts enabled us to orient the temporal bone in an accurate anatomical position on the tomographic table.

Schuknecht (1958) has detailed the procedure for obtaining temporal bones, and we followed his suggestions, including ligature of the internal carotid artery.

Upon removal, we placed the bones in 10% formalin for preservation until the time of the tomographic study.

We sectioned each bone tomographically in one of the six planes described below.

Preliminary tomographs were made and the position of the bone on the x-ray table was adjusted until the desired anatomical plane was obtained. Sections 1mm apart were obtained throughout the entire thickness of the bone.

Since the plane of tomographic sectioning was parallel to the table top, each bone was marked with india ink circumferentially in a horizontal plane. This india ink line was our guide for the macrosectioning.

Each bone was decalcified in 2.5% nitric acid for approximately three weeks. The decalcification was monitored radiographically. Just as the last bit of calcium disappeared from the bone, the decalcification was stopped.

The bones were then placed in 10% formalin for two to three weeks to harden the tissue and facilitate macrosectioning.

A commercial meat slicer was used for the macrosections. Meat slicers have been previously used for macrosectioning of the lung and other structures.

We found that we could section the human temporal bone easily and quickly with this type of meat slicer. Since the slicer cuts and does not saw, there is no loss of tissue, except of the occasional loss of minute bits of the ossicles which were separated from all their attachments. The meat slicer is sharp enough to bisect the long process of the incus longitudinally.

The 2 mm thick macrosections were stored in 10% formalin until ready for photography.

Using a macro photography setup, each side of each bone was photographed at 1:1 magnification. For the illustrations in this atlas we used Kodachrome film. For preparatory study of the bones, we made Kodachrome transparencies and projected them.

We made microradiographs of each section using the method described on pp. 3,4.

With the Kodachrome transparencies of the surfaces of the sections, the tomographs, and the microradiographs, we were able to examine and compare each section by three different methods.

We sectioned approximately 125 temporal bones. For presentation in this atlas we selected for each projection one normal bone in which the planes of the macrosections and the tomograms coincided as exactly as possible. We have also included selected macosections and radiographs from nine of the pathologic temporal bones we encountered in our study.

The 2 mm thick tissue macrosections have three dimensions, two surfaces and the intervening 2 mm thick layer of tissue. The tomographs and microradiographs help in visualizing fine structures not seen on the surface of the section which may be included within the 2 mm thickness.

Because there is no loss of tissue using the knife of the meat slicer, we were able to restack the tissue sections carefully under precise microscopic control and reconstruct the entire block of the bone rather easily. Reconstruction of the temporal bone from histologic sections is a complicated and time-consuming process.

Using a 1:1 photographic setup and Kodachrome film,

we photographed the reconstructed temporal bone and took serial photographs as each 2 mm thick section was removed.

We photographed the serial dissection of the block from the two aspects. For the coronal sections, for instance, we photographed the anterior aspect of the block serially after removal of each section. We then reconstructed the bone and photographed the block from the posterior aspect, again serially, after removal of each separate section. When we mounted these photographs serially in the automatic projector we were able to view the anatomy of the bone, in an anterior or posterior dissection, as section after section was removed. By reversing the projector we achieved the effect of reconstructing the block.

In this manner we were able to "bisect" the reconstructed tissue block at 10 to 14 different planes throughout the temporal bone.

For the study of specific areas and structures of the temporal bone, we were able to appose two or three sections quickly and easibly and obtain "instant" reconstruction at any desired level.

We have not included any of the block reconstructions in the illustrations of this book, although we worked out many anatomical details by using this method.

When it was necessary to study the temporal bone histologically we found that we could process a 2 mm thick section of temporal bone with the usual celloidin method and obtain 25 μ thick histologic sections.

Figures 9.113 and 10.20 are examples of photomicrographs of histological sections made from two macrosections. Figure 9.113 is from the macrosection in Fig. 9.88 and 9.90 and shows a small epitympanic cholesteatoma. Figure 10.20 shows the histopathology of otosclerosis in the bone studied in Chapter 10.

In most laboratories temporal bones are sectioned either through the horizontal plane or through an axial plane. Using the present technique we have varied the plane of section through six planes: horizontal, coronal, semiaxial, axial, sagittal, and the longitudinal (Stenvers) plane.

When we encountered a temporal bone with pathologic findings, we tomographed the bone in several planes to discover which plane demonstrated the pathology best, and to decide which plane would be most advantageous for macrosectioning.

With the tomographs we established the desired plane, marked the bone, and cut along this plane.

In this atlas we have reversed the second surface of each section for better understanding and correlation of the tissue sections with the tomographs and microradiographs. Each reversed section is so marked to avoid confusion.

Thus, for example, in the 2 mm thick section of the right temporal bone cut in the horizontal plane, in Fig. 2.1–2.7, the superior surface of the section in Fig. 2.3 is reproduced as a section of a *right* temporal bone. The inferior surface of this same section, Fig. 2.5, is reproduced photographically as if it were the inferior surface of a *left* temporal bone.

In some sections, the spatial relationships of the structures are altered somewhat by presenting the second surface of the bone in the reversed position. However, we feel that this reversal aids in the correlation with the radiographs.

Microradiography of the Temporal Bone

Microradiography is a high-definition technique using soft x-rays for the study of soft tissue specimens and thin sections of calcified specimens.

In this study, a microradiograph of each decalcified 2 mm thick macrosection was obtained. We employed a Faxitron model 804 machine which has a beryllium window in the x-ray tube transmitting low voltage x-rays with minimum attenuation. This allows good contrast of low density structures. The factors were the following: focus film distance 13.9 inches voltage 15 Kv, exposure time 15 seconds. Kodak MA 2 mammography films were used which were processed in a medical automatic processor. Since the tissue sections were placed directly on the paper wrapping of the film there was practically no magnification nor geometrical distortion of the structures included in the 2 mm thick tissue slices.

The application of microradiography to study macrosections was extremely interesting, since the system represents an intermediate method of examination between tomography and photography. The microradiograph includes all the details of an ideal tomographic section. The microradiograph also resembles the photographs of the section, since it shows the soft tissue structures which are visible on the two surfaces of each section. Because of the nature of the penetrating x-rays, the microradiographs add depth to the visualization of the macrosections. Microradiographs show anatomical features of the entire thickness of the tissue, including structures hidden within the slice. These hidden structures are not visualized microscopically or in the photographs of the surfaces of the macrosections. The low kilovoltage technique used in microradiography permits visualization of practically all the tissue in the section including portions of the membranous labyrinth, ossicular ligaments and tympanic membrane. Unlike the tomographs, microradiographs are obtained from decalcified bones. Therefore, the decalcified osteoid and the soft tissue structures included in the section have the same coefficient of absorption of the x-rays and the same radiographic density. For this reason, the facial nerve canal is poorly visualized in the microradiographs, since the contour of the decalcified bony canal is obliterated by the similar density of the enclosed nerve.

The difference in densities seen in the microradiographs depends not on the degree of ossification, but only on the thickness of the various structures.

Tomographic Projections of the Temporal Bone

The criteria we have followed in the selection of tomographic projections are: 1) the projection should be easy to obtain and reproduce at a later date should

repeat tomography be necessary; 2) the projection should section the structures of the ear at an angle which gives optimal visualization; 3) if possible, the tomographic section should follow the planes of surgical approach or histological sectioning familiar to the otologist.

Six different radiographic projections and planes of section were used in this study: 1) coronal or frontal; 2) sagittal or lateral; 3) horizontal or basal; 4) semiaxial of the petrous pyramid or 20° coronal oblique of the skull; 5) longitudinal of the petrous pyramid or Stenvers; 6) axial of the petrous pyramid or Pöschle.

In the first two projections, the terms coronal and sagittal refer to planes of the skull and not to planes of the petrous pyramid, since the pyramids are actually sectioned in both views at 45° to the long axis. In the horizontal projection, the horizontal planes of the skull and of the petrous pyramids coincide. In the Stenvers and axial projections, the term longitudinal and axial refer to the long axis of the petrous pyramid.

In clinical work it is preferable to use external landmarks to orient the skull when obtaining a certain radiographic projection.

References

Anson, B.J., J.A.Donaldson: The Surgical Anatomy of the Temporal Bone and Ear. Saunders, Philadelphia 1967

Bast, T.H., B.J.Anson: The Temporal Bone and the Ear. Charles C.Thomas, Springfield 1949

Buckingham, R.A., G.E.Valvassori: Tomographic and Surgical Pathology of Cholesteatoma. Arch. Otolaryng. 91: 464–469, 1970

Compere, W.E.: Radiographic Atlas of the Temporal Bone, Vol. 1. American Academy of Ophthalmology and Otolaryngology, Rochester, 1964

Mündnich, K., K.-W.Frey: The Tomogram of the Ear. Thieme, Stuttgart 1959

Schuknecht, H.: Technique for acquiring and preparing the human temporal bone for pathological study and for anatomical-surgical dissection. Trans. Amer. Acad. Ophthal. 62: 601, 1958

Shambaugh, G.E., Jr.: Surgery of the Ear, Second Edition. Saunders, Philadelphia 1967

Spalteholz, W., trans. by L.F.Barker: Hand-Atlas of Human Anatomy, Vol. III. Lippincott, Philadelphia 1943

Valvassori, G.E.: Radiographic Atlas of the Temporal Bone, Vol. II. American Academy of Ophthalmology and Otolaryngology, Rochester 1964

Valvassori, G.E., R.H.Pierce: The normal internal auditory canal. Amer. J. Roentgenol. 92: 1232–2141, 1964

Valvassori, G.E.: Otosclerosis: A new challenge to roentgenology. Amer. J. Roentgenol. Radiol. Therap. 94: 566–575, 1965

Valvassori, G.E.: The interpretation of the radiographic findings in cochlear otosclerosis. Ann. Otol. (St.Louis) 75: 572–578, 1966

Valvassori, G.E.: The abnormal internal auditory canal: The diagnosis of acoustic neuroma. Radiology 92, 449–459, 1969a

Valvassori, G.E., R.F.Naunton, J.R.Lindsay: Inner ear anomalies: Clinical and histopathological considerations. Ann. Otol. (St.Louis) 78: 929–938, 1969b

Valvassori, G.E., R.A.Buckingham: Microradiography and macrosectioning of the temporal bone. Ann. Otol. (St.Louis) 79: 1–5, 1970

Valvassori, G.E.: In: Radiography of the Temporal Bone in Otolaryngology, Vol. 1. ed. by: M.M. Paparella and D.A. Shumrick. Saunders, Philadelphia 1973

Wolff, D., R.J.Bellucci, A.Eggston: Microscopic Anatomy of the Temporal Bone. Williams and Wilkins, Baltimore 1957

The Normal Temporal Bone

Chapter 2   Horizontal Projection and Horizontal Sections

The horizontal projection is quite satisfactory for the study of the temporal bone, especially of the petrous portion. Unfortunately, it is very uncomfortable for the patient to maintain his head in a satisfactory position for the length of the study, and with the horizontal projection it is difficult to reproduce identical views at a later date. We use this view in fractures and tumors of the temporal bone. In selected cases, this view is useful in visualizing the extension of a lesion to the adjacent floor of the middle and posterior cranial fossae.

The horizontal projection is obtained in the submentovertex direction. The patient is supine with the back elevated from the table with some kind of support and the head overextended until the vertex touches the table top (Fig. 2.1).

In this atlas the isolated temporal bones were positioned with the superior surface of the petrous pyramid parallel to the plane of the film.

Six consecutive sections of a normal right temporal bone are shown, each 2 mm thick. The photographs of the inferior aspect of each section have been reversed to facilitate comparison with the corresponding tomograms and microradiographs which are included.

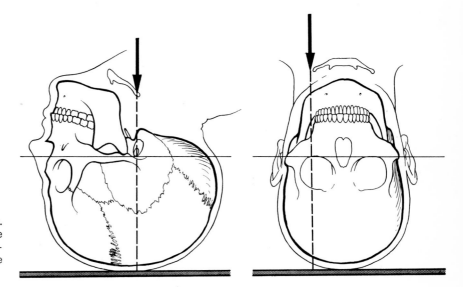

2.1 Horizontal projection, head position. The orbitomeatal plane is parallel to the film plane. The arrows indicate the position of the centering point on the surface of the head.

Horizontal Sections

Figures 2.2–2.7 expose the structures in a 2 mm thick horizontal section of a right, adult temporal bone, 2 mm inferior to the arcuate eminence.

The mastoid air cells occupy the lateral portion of the section; the anterior and posterior limbs of the superior semicircular canal are in the center. Subarcuate vessels pass between the limbs of the superior canal.

The superior petrosal sinus courses along the superior margin of the petrous apex.

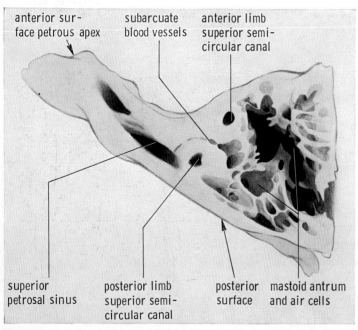

2.2 Drawing of structures seen in Fig. 2.3 to 2.7.

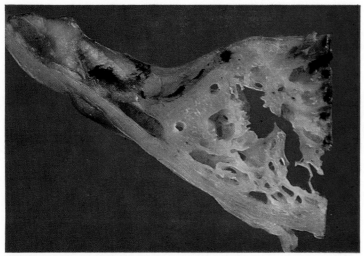

2.3 Photograph of superior surface of an horizontal macrosection two mm below the arcuate eminence.

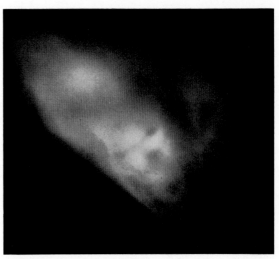

2.4 Tomograph corresponding to Fig. 2.3.

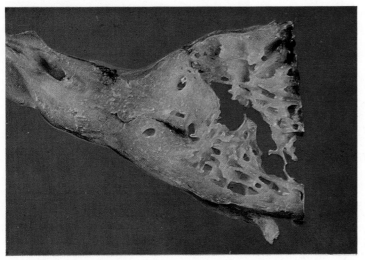

2.5 Photograph of inferior surface of horizontal macrosection Fig. 2.3. Reversed photographically.

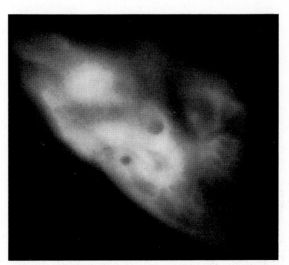

2.6 Tomograph corresponding to Fig. 2.5.

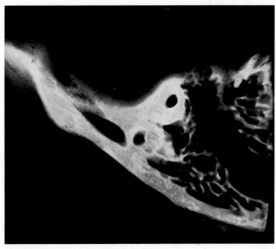

2.7 Microradiograph of macrosection seen in Fig. 2.3 and 2.5.

Horizontal Sections

Figures 2.8–2.13 show the structures in a 2 mm thick horizontal section of a right adult temporal bone immediately inferior to Fig. 2.2–2.7.

The aditus of the mastoid antrum opens into the epitympanum. Mastoid air cells surround the epitympanum and antrum.

Superior portions of the malleus head and incus body appear in the epitympanum.

The nonampullated limbs of the superior and posterior semicircular canals join at the crus commune.

The subarcuate vessels pass from the subarcuate fossa laterally between the limbs of the superior semicircular canal.

On the inferior surface of the tissue section, the horizontal semicircular canal forms the medial wall of the antrum, and the ampullated portions of the horizontal and superior semicircular canals open into the superior portion of the vestibule. This surface also exposes the roof of the internal auditory canal and two small branches of the facial nerve in the region of the geniculate ganglion (Fig. 2.11 and 2.12).

The shadow of the cochlea appears in the tomographs anterior to the fundus of the internal auditory canal (Fig. 2.12).

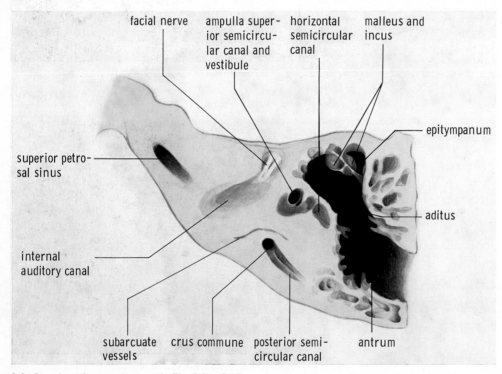

2.8 Drawing of structures seen in Fig. 2.9 to 2.13.

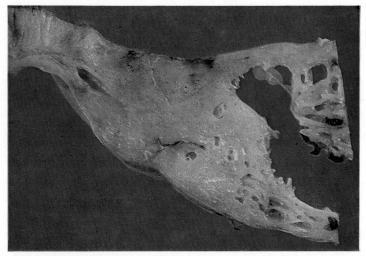

2.9 Photograph of superior surface of the horizontal macrosection immediately inferior to Fig. 2.5.

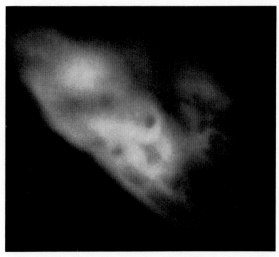

2.10 Tomograph corresponding to Fig. 2.9.

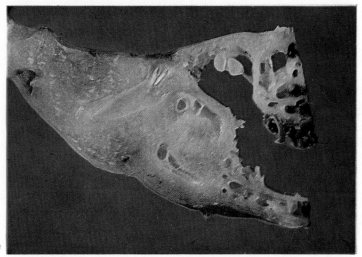

2.11 Photograph of inferior surface of horizontal macrosection Fig. 2.9. Reversed photographically.

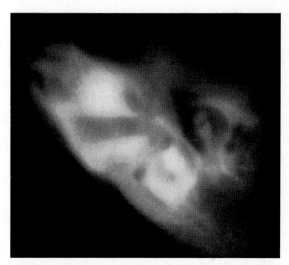

2.12 Tomograph corresponding to Fig. 2.11.

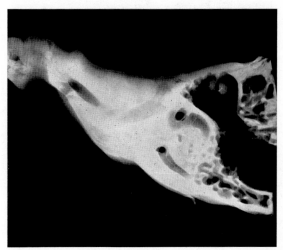

2.13 Microradiograph of macrosection seen in Fig. 2.9 and 2.11.

Horizontal Sections

Figures 2.14–2.19 reveal the structures in a 2 mm thick horizontal section of a right adult temporal bone immediately inferior to Fig. 2.8–2.13.

Mastoid air cells surround the antrum and extend lateral to the epitympanum. The malleus head and incus body occupy the epitympanum, and the incus short process rests in the fossa incudis.

The cavity of the epitympanum assumes a somewhat triangular shape at this level. The medial and lateral epitympanic walls converge posteriorly at the aditus, while the base of the triangle lies anterior. The medial wall forms a 20° to 25° angle with the sagittal plane crossing the fossa incudis. The lateral wall forms a 10° angle lateral to the sagittal plane at the fossa incudis.

The ampullated end of the horizontal semicircular canal enters the vestibule anterior on the superior surface of the section, Fig. 2.15 and 2.16, and the nonampullated end opens into the posterior portion of the vestibule on the inferior surface of the section (Fig. 2.17, 2.18).

The posterior semicircular canal extends posterolaterally from the crus commune.

The macula of the utricle stretches across the upper portion of the vestibule (Fig. 2.17).

The facial and superior vestibular nerves occupy the internal auditory canal.

The superior vestibular nerve arches towards the utricular macula and the ampullae of the horizontal and superior semicircular canals.

The petrous portion of the facial nerve extends from the internal auditory canal to the geniculate ganglion (Fig. 2.15). At the geniculate ganglion the nerve turns sharply into the horizontal position and extends posterior along the medial wall of the tympanum just below the horizontal semicircular canal (Fig. 2.17, 2.18). Superior portions of the basal and middle coils of the cochlea appear anterior to the fundus of the internal auditory canal.

The superior turn of the vestibular aqueduct passes adjacent to the posterior semicircular canal on the inferior surface of the section (Fig. 2.17, 2.19).

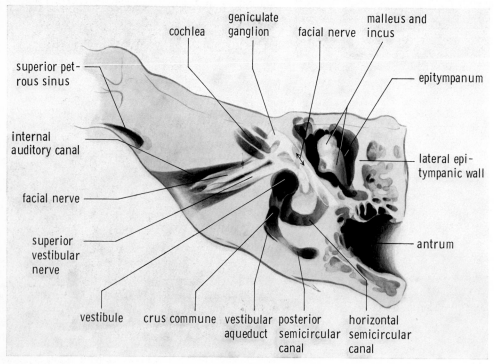

2.14 Drawing of structures seen in Fig. 2.15 to 2.19.

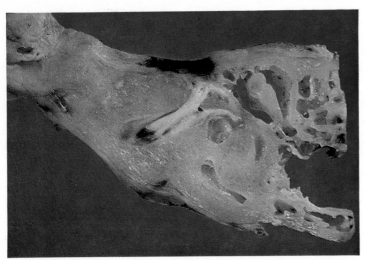

2.15 Photograph of superior surface of the horizontal macrosection imme-diately inferior to Fig. 2.11.

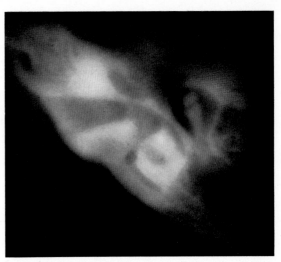

2.16 Tomograph corresponding to Fig. 2.15.

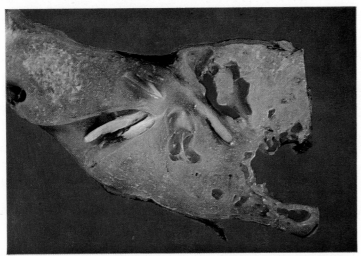

2.17 Photograph of inferior surface of horizontal macrosection Fig. 2.15. Reversed photographically.

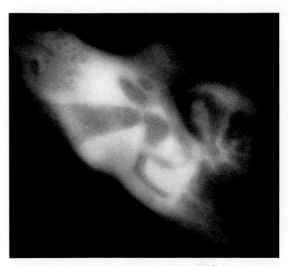

2.18 Tomograph corresponding to Fig. 2.17.

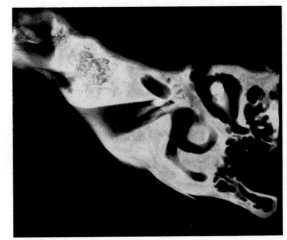

2.19 Microradiograph of macrosection seen in Fig. 2.15 and 2.17.

Horizontal Sections

Figures 2.20–2.25 demonstrate the structures in a 2 mm thick horizontal section of a right adult temporal bone immediately inferior to Fig. 2.14–2.19.

The section crosses the mastoid antrum and the superior wall of the external auditory canal.

The tendon of the tensor tympani muscle stretches from the cochleariform process to the neck of the malleus. The tensor muscle appears on the inferior surface of the section (Fig. 2.23).

In the oval window, the outer surface of the stapes footplate is canted slightly downwards and the incudostapedial joint lies slightly below the level of the footplate.

The facial nerve extends from the oval window to the second turn.

On the inferior surface of the section, the stapedius tendon and the pyramidal eminence lie anteromedial to the facial nerve (Fig. 2.23).

The stapes footplate at this level forms the lateral wall of the vestibule. The membranous ampullated end of the posterior semicircular canal joins the utricle on the posteromedial margin of the vestibule (Fig. 2.23).

The nerve to the ampulla of the posterior semicircular canal leaves the internal auditory canal at the foramen singulare (Fig. 2.23).

The posterior semicircular canal lies anterior to the vestibular aqueduct. At this level the endolymphatic sac enters the vestibular aqueduct (Fig. 2.25).

The section passes through the modiolus and three turns of the cochlea.

In the internal auditory canal, the cochlear nerve turns anteriorly into the modiolus 2–3 mm medial to the fundus of the canal.

The cochlear and inferior vestibular nerves lie in the inferior compartment of the internal auditory canal.

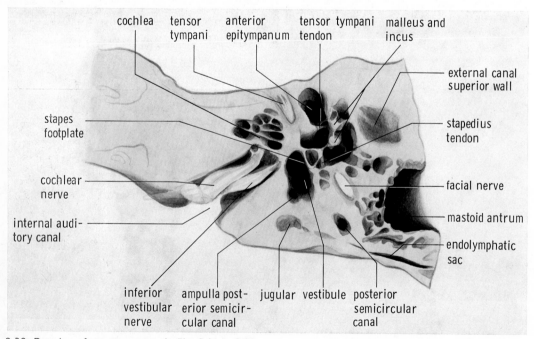

2.20 Drawing of structures seen in Fig. 2.21 to 2.25.

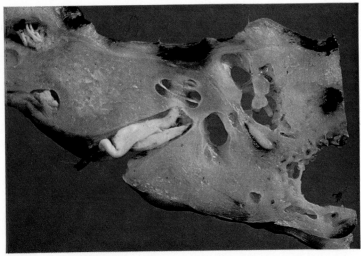

2.21 Photograph of superior surface of the horizontal macrosection immediately inferior to Fig. 2.17.

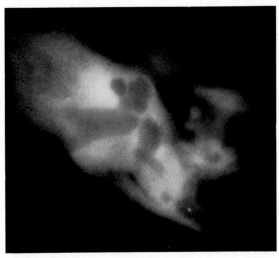

2.22 Tomograph corresponding to Fig. 2.21.

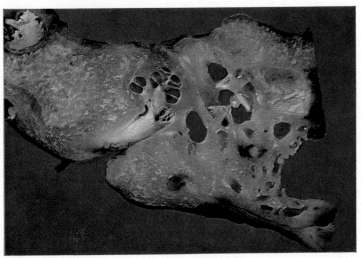

2.23 Photograph of inferior surface of horizontal macrosection Fig. 2.21. Reversed photographically.

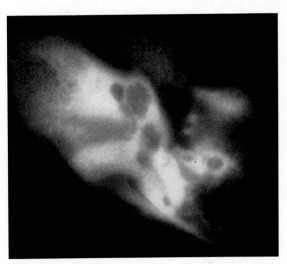

2.24 Tomograph corresponding to Fig. 2.23.

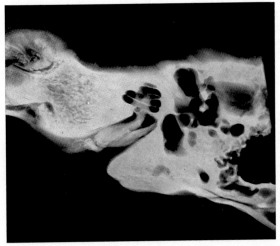

2.25 Microradiograph of macrosection seen in Fig. 2.21 and 2.23.

Horizontal Sections

Figures 2.26–2.31 show the structures in a 2 mm thick horizontal section of a right adult temporal bone immediately inferior to Fig. 2.20–2.25.

A section of the tympanic membrane with a portion of the malleus handle separates the external canal from the middle ear.

The lenticular process lies just posterior to the malleus handle. The tensor tympani canal lies on the anterior portion of the medial wall of the middle ear. The descending portion of the facial nerve lies in the posterior wall of the middle ear lateral to the pyramidal eminence and to the tympanic sinus.

The proximal portion of the basal coil of the cochlea forms the promontory of the medial wall of the middle ear. All three coils of the cochlea appear on the superior surface of the section (Fig. 2.27, 2.28). Only the basal coil remains on the inferior surface (Fig. 2.29, 2.30).

The spiral lamina separates the scala vestibuli from the scala tympani. In the niche of the round window, the round window membrane closes the scala tympani. At the fundus of the internal auditory canal, small twigs of the cochlear nerve supply part of the basal turn.

The ampulla of the posterior semicircular canal, as it enters the inferior and posterior portion of the vestibule lies close to the round window. The posterior semicircular canal arches posterior within the thickness of the tissue section between the facial canal anterior and the endolymphatic sac posterior.

The dome of the jugular fossa lies at the anteromedial margin of the endolymphatic sac.

The cochlear aqueduct passes medially from the round window area on the inferior surface of the section (Fig. 2.29, 2.31).

The carotid artery appears anterior to the basal turn of the cochlea.

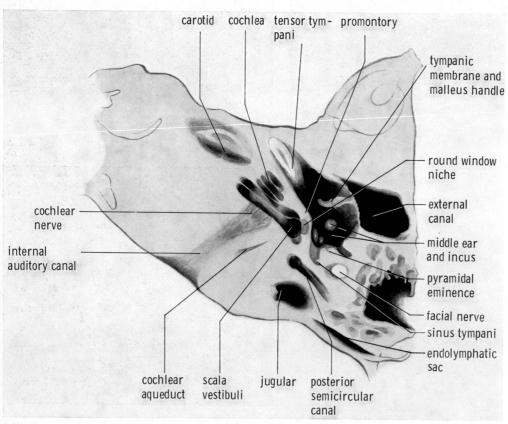

2.26 Drawing of structures seen in Fig. 2.27 to 2.31.

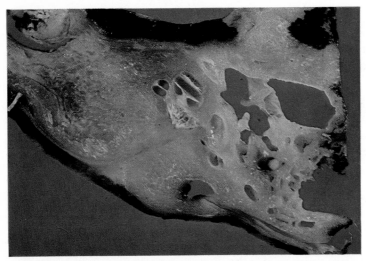

2.27 Photograph of superior surface of the horizontal macrosection immediately inferior to Fig. 2.23.

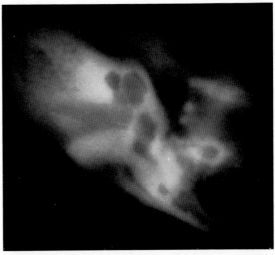

2.28 Tomograph corresponding to Fig. 2.27.

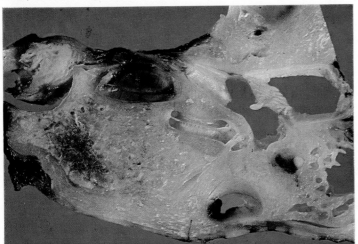

2.29 Photograph of inferior surface of horizontal macrosection Fig. 2.27. Reversed photographically.

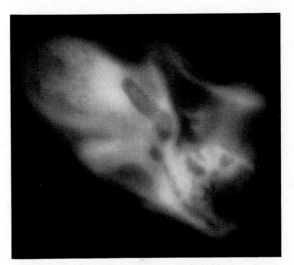

2.30 Tomograph corresponding to Fig. 2.29.

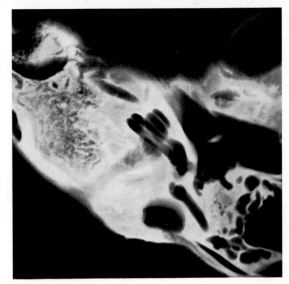

2.31 Microradiograph of macrosection seen in Fig. 2.27 and 2.29.

Horizontal Sections

Figures 2.32–2.37 reveal the structures in a 2 mm thick horizontal section of a right adult temporal bone immediately inferior to Fig. 2.26–2.31.

The tip of the malleus handle lies in the umbo in a strip of the tympanic membrane. The tensor tympani muscle lies lateral to the internal carotid artery.

The eustachian tube extends anteriorly under the tensor tympani muscle (Fig. 2.35).

The descending facial nerve lies lateral to the jugular fossa.

The inferior portion of the basal turn of the cochlea bounds the medial wall of the middle ear (Fig. 2.33).

The cochlear aqueduct lies medial to the jugular fossa and widens as it opens into the subarachnoid space.

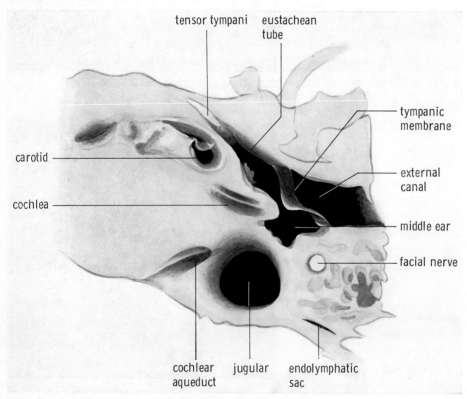

2.32   Drawing of structures seen in Fig. 2.33 to 2.37.

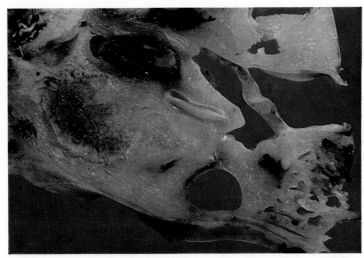

2.33 Photograph of superior surface of the horizontal macrosection immediately inferior to Fig. 2.29.

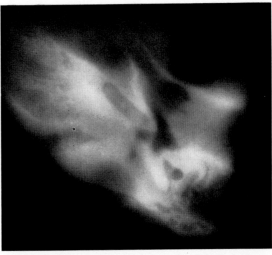

2.34 Tomograph corresponding to Fig. 2.33.

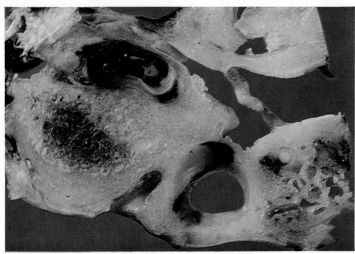

2.35 Photograph of inferior surface of horizontal macrosection Fig. 2.33. Reversed photographically.

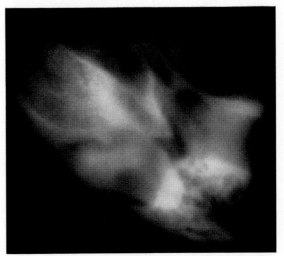

2.36 Tomograph corresponding to Fig. 2.35.

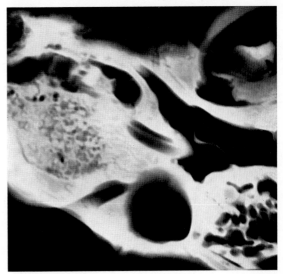

2.37 Microradiograph of macrosection seen in Fig. 2.33 and 2.35.

Chapter 3   Coronal Projection and Coronal Sections

The coronal projection is quite satisfactory for the study of all three portions of the ear, comfortable for the patient and easy to obtain and reproduce. We consider it a basic projection, and we use it in all instances except for the study of the vestibular aqueduct.

The coronal projection is obtained with the patient supine, or occasionally prone. The plane from the tragus to the outer canthus of the eye is perpendicular to the plane of the film. When it is necessary to obtain good visualization of the tegmen tympani, which slopes downward anterior, the patient's chin should be extended until the plane from the tragus to the inferior orbital rim becomes perpendicular to the film (Fig. 3.1).

For this atlas, the isolated temporal bones were positioned with the long axis of the petrous pyramid at 45° to the plane of the film.

Seven consecutive tissue sections of the left temporal bone are shown. Each section is 2 mm thick. Corresponding tomographs, 1 mm apart, and microradiographs of each tissue section are included. To facilitate the comparison with the tomograms and microradiographs, the photograph of the posterior aspect of each tissue section has been reversed and shown in the same orientation as the photograph of the anterior aspect of the tissue section.

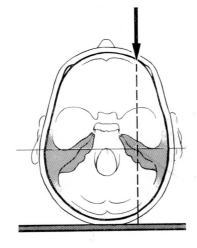 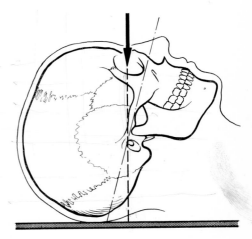

3.1   Coronal projection, head position. The coronal plane of the skull is parallel to the film plane. A line from the outer canthus to the tragus is perpendicular to the film plane. The arrows indicate the position of the centering point on the surface of the head.

Coronal Sections

Figures 3.2–3.7 expose the structures in a 2 mm thick coronal section of a left adult temporal bone at the level of the anterior wall of the external auditory canal, the most anterior portion of the tympanic membrane, and the posterior aspect of the temporomandibular joint.

A small slice of the anterior portion of the malleus head appears in the epitympanum. A thin bony septum separates the hypotympanum from the carotid canal.

The geniculate ganglion of the facial nerve lies above the cochlea, while the tensor tympani canal lies on the medial wall of the middle ear.

The radiographic appearance of the cochlea is caused by the radiolucency of the modiolus and the bony spiral lamina. Thus the tomograms show only the wall and lumen of the spiral cochlear canal and the septa that separate the basal, middle and apical coils.

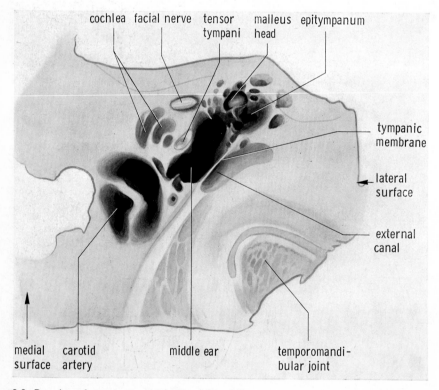

3.2 Drawing of structures seen in Fig. 3.3 to 3.7.

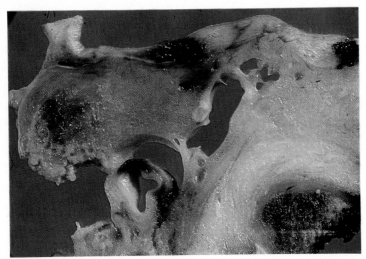

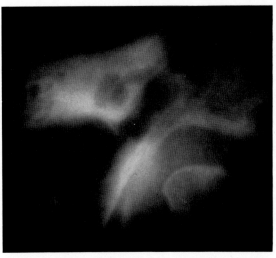

3.3 Photograph of anterior surface of a coronal macrosection at the level anterior wall of the external auditory canal.

3.4 Tomograph corresponding to Fig. 3.3.

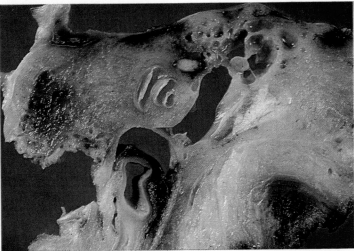

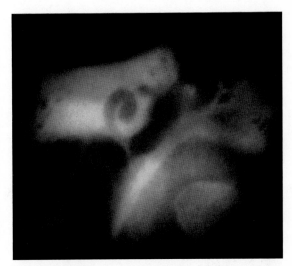

3.5 Photograph of posterior surface of coronal macrosection Fig. 3.3. Reversed photographically.

3.6 Tomograph corresponding to Fig. 3.5.

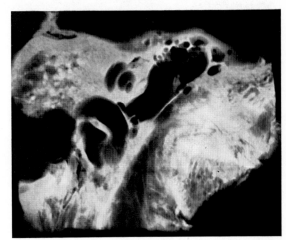

3.7 Microradiograph of macrosection seen in Fig. 3.3 and 3.5.

Coronal Sections

Figures 3.8–3.13 demonstrate the structures present in a 2 mm thick coronal section of a left adult temporal bone, immediately posterior to Fig. 3.2–3.7.

A thin section of tympanic membrane divides the external auditory canal from the middle ear. A small area of the pars flaccida is retracted above the mallear short process in the notch of Rivinus. The tendon of the tensor tympani stretches across the middle ear from the cochleariform process to the mallear neck.

The lateral wall of the epitympanum joins the superior wall of the external auditory canal in a sharp edge lateral to the malleus neck.

A portion of the body of the incus projects laterally from the articulation with the malleus head. This accounts for the characteristic bilobed appearance of the ossicular mass in the tomographs.

Within the thickness of the tissue section, the facial nerve bifurcates from the geniculate ganglion into the petrous and tympanic segments. In the tomograms this bifurcation appears as paired, adjacent, circular foramina.

Portions of the basal, middle, and apical coils of the cochlea lie superior to the carotid canal.

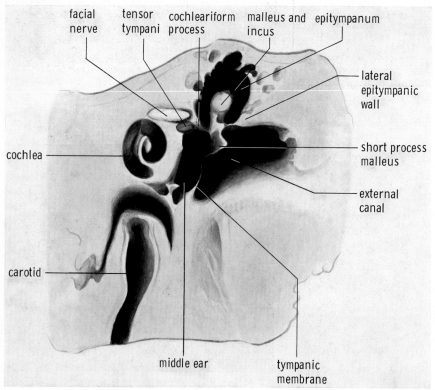

3.8 Drawing of structures seen in Fig. 3.9 to 3.13.

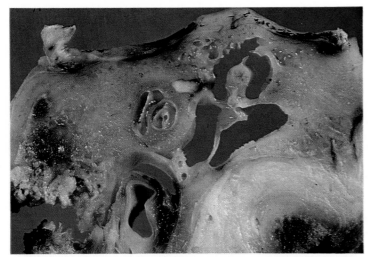

3.9   Photograph of anterior surface of the coronal macrosection immediately posterior to Fig. 3.5.

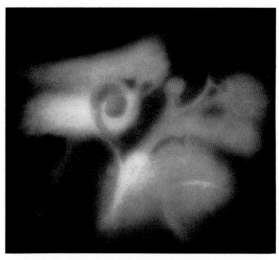

3.10   Tomograph corresponding to Fig. 3.9.

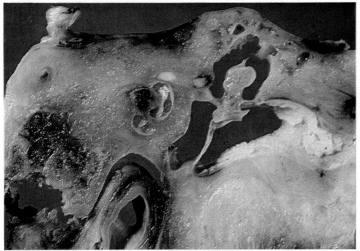

3.11   Photograph of posterior surface of coronal macrosection Fig. 3.9. Reversed photographically.

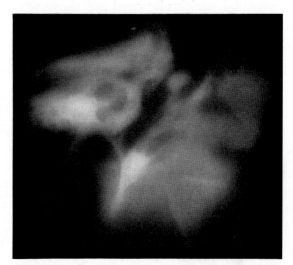

3.12   Tomograph corresponding to Fig. 3.11.

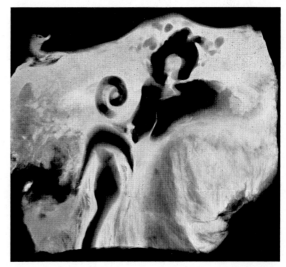

3.13   Microradiograph of macrosection seen in Fig. 3.9 and 3.11.

Coronal Sections

Figures 3.14–3.19 demonstrate the structures in a 2 mm thick coronal section of a left adult temporal bone immediately posterior to Fig. 3.8–3.13.

The tympanic membrane with the malleus handle attached separates the external canal from the middle ear.

The inferior margin of the lateral attic wall and the superior wall of the external canal form a triangular projection with the apex directed medially.

Portions of the body and long process of the incus lie in the epitympanum between the prominence of the horizontal semicircular canal and the lateral epitympanic wall.

The tympanic portion of the facial nerve lies below the horizontal semicircular canal and above the anterior margin of the oval window. A small anterior portion of the stapes footplate and anterior crus are in the oval window. The proximal portion of the facial nerve lies in the upper compartment of the internal auditory canal.

The posterior surface of the tissue section (Fig. 3.17), reveals the anterior wall of the vestibule, the horizontal and superior semicircular canals, and the internal auditory canal. Portions of the membranous labyrinth are present within the lumina of the vestibule and semicircular canals.

Below the facial nerve, the cochlear nerve enters the foraminous spiral tract of the modiolus.

The proximal part of the basal coil of the cochlea forms the promontory of the medial wall of the middle ear. The carotid artery lies inferiorly.

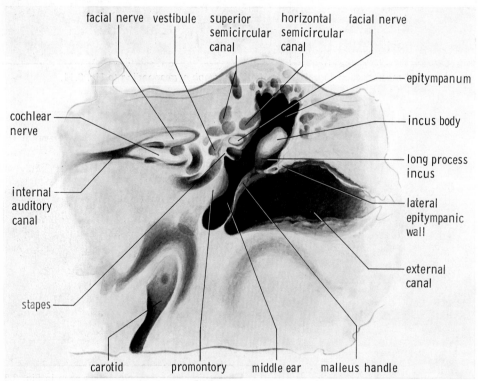

3.14 Drawing of structures seen in Fig. 3.15 to 3.19.

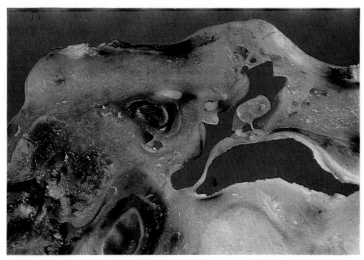

3.15 Photograph of anterior surface of the coronal macrosection immediately posterior to Fig. 3.11.

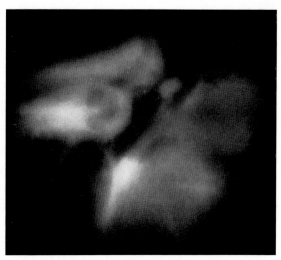

3.16 Tomograph corresponding to Fig. 3.15.

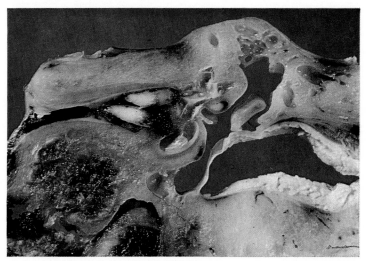

3.17 Photograph of posterior surface of coronal macrosection Fig. 3.15. Reversed photographically.

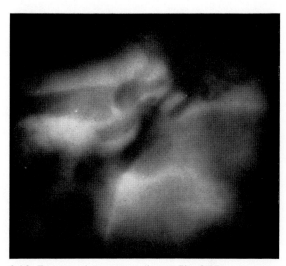

3.18 Tomograph corresponding to Fig. 3.17.

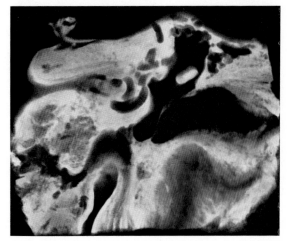

3.19 Microradiograph of macrosection seen in Fig. 3.15 and 3.17.

Coronal Sections

Figures 3.20–3.25 show the structure in a 2 mm thick coronal section of a left adult temporal bone immediately posterior to Fig. 3.14–3.19.

The tympanic membrane separates the external and middle ears.

The long process of the incus extends to the stapes. A portion of the long process is missing in the tissue section (Fig. 3.21). On the posterior surface of the tissue section, the tip of the short process of the incus lies in the aditus between the lateral epitympanic wall and the prominence of the horizontal semicircular canal (Fig. 3.23). The mastoid antrum extends superior and posterior from the aditus.

The section exposes the vestibule and the ampullated portions of the superior and horizontal semicircular canals. The utricle and the macula of the utricle occupy the upper portion of the bony vestibule. A portion of the saccule lies on the medial vestibular wall.

The facial nerve appears between the horizontal semicircular canal and the oval window. This section includes most of the stapes footplate and superstructure.

The scala vestibuli opens into the inferior portion of the vestibule, while the scala tympani extends to the round window. The round window lies on the posterior and inferior surface of the promontory (Fig. 3.23). Mucosal folds obscure the round window niche and membrane. In the tomographs the round window niche appears as a dehiscence in the contour of the inferior basal turn.

There are segments of the facial and acoustic cranial nerves in the internal auditory canal.

Hypotympanic air cells extend inferior from the mesotympanum.

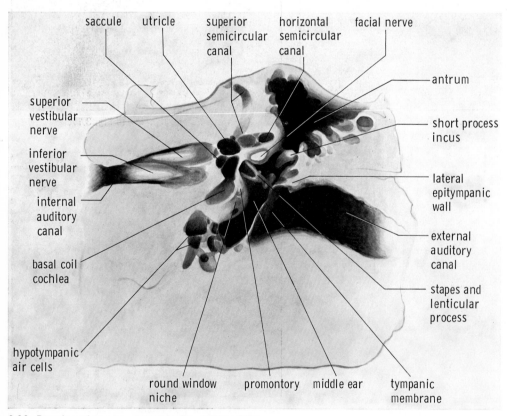

3.20 Drawing of structures seen in Fig. 3.21 to 3.25.

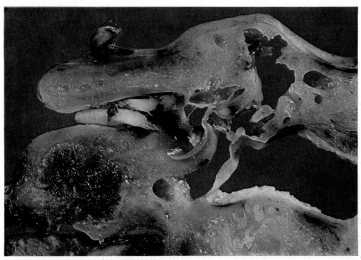

3.21 Photograph of anterior surface of the coronal macrosection imme-diately posterior to Fig. 3.17.

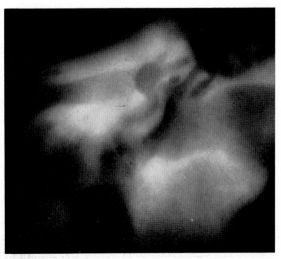

3.22 Tomograph corresponding to Fig. 3.21.

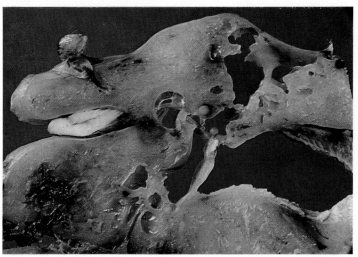

3.23 Photograph of posterior surface of coronal macrosection Fig. 3.21. Reversed photographically.

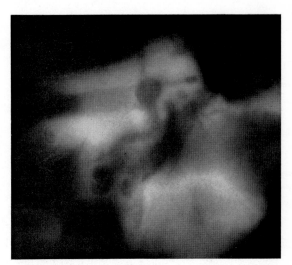

3.24 Tomograph corresponding to Fig. 3.23.

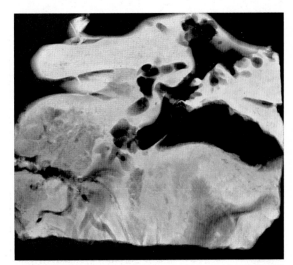

3.25 Microradiograph of macrosection seen in Fig. 3.21 and 3.23.

Coronal Sections

Figures 3.26–3.31 reveal the structures in a 2 mm thick coronal section of a left adult temporal bone immediately posterior to Figs. 3.20–3.25.

The section exposes the posterior wall of the external auditory canal, a small portion of the tympanic membrane, and the posterior portion of the middle ear.

The horizontal semicircular canal protrudes into the mastoid antrum.

The superior semicircular canal joins the crus commune above the vestibule.

The facial nerve lies inferior to the horizontal semicircular canal. The pyramidal eminence with the tendon of the stapedius muscle is below the facial nerve. The extension of the middle ear medial to the pyramidal eminence represents the sinus tympani.

The facial recess lies between the facial nerve and the posterosuperior portion of the tympanic membrane. The ampullated end of the posterior semicircular canal opens into the inferior portion of the vestibule on the posterior surface of the section (Fig. 3.29). A remnant of the round window niche appears on the anterior surface of the section at the same level (Fig. 3.27).

The posterior wall of the internal auditory canal is present.

The cochlear aqueduct stretches inferior from the round window area to the jugular foramen.

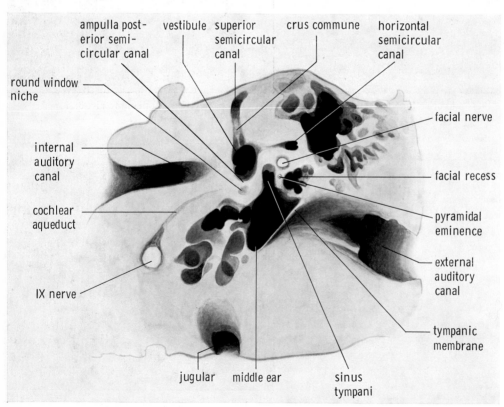

3.26 Drawing of structures seen in Fig. 3.27 to 3.31.

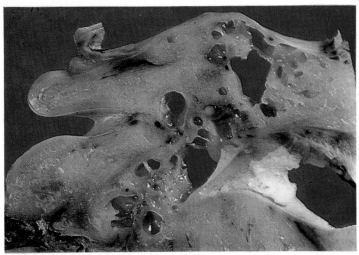

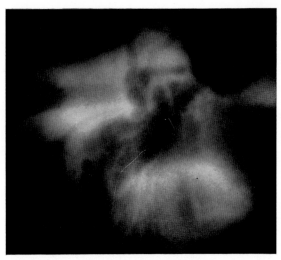

3.27 Photograph of anterior surface of the coronal macrosection immediately posterior to Fig. 3.23.

3.28 Tomograph corresponding to Fig. 3.27.

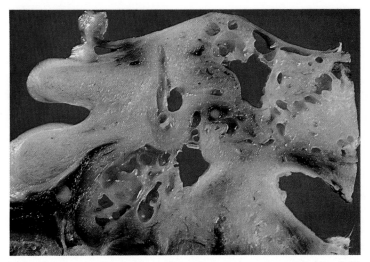

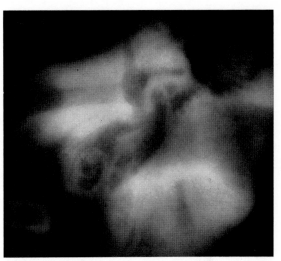

3.29 Photograph of posterior surface of coronal macrosection Fig. 3.27.
Reversed photographically.

3.30 Tomograph corresponding to Fig. 3.29.

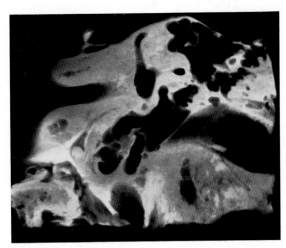

3.31 Microradiograph of macrosection seen in Fig. 3.27
and 3.29.

Coronal Sections

Figures 3.32–3.37 show the structures in a 2 mm thick coronal section of a left adult temporal bone immediately posterior to Figs. 3.26–3.31.

The section passes through the posterior wall of the external auditory canal and mastoid air cells.

The posterior limb of the horizontal semicircular canal bulges into the mastoid antrum.

The crus commune, the posterior limb of the horizontal semicircular canal, and the ampulla of the posterior semicircular canal open into the posterior portion of the vestibule.

Portions of the membranous labyrinth are present within the bony canals (Fig. 3.33).

The pyramidal turn of the facial nerve lies under the horizontal semicircular canal.

Air cells extend posteriorly and medially from the posterior wall of the middle ear.

The jugular opening of the cochlear aqueduct lies between the porus of the internal auditory canal and the jugular fossa.

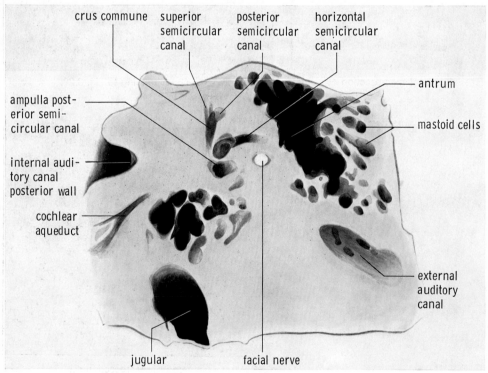

3.32   Drawing of structures seen in Fig. 3.33 to 3.37.

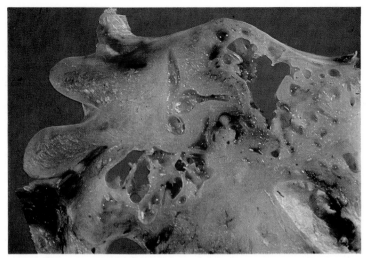

3.33 Photograph of anterior surface of the coronal macrosection immediately posterior to Fig. 3.29.

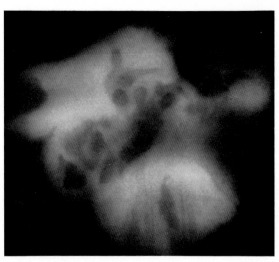

3.34 Tomograph corresponding to Fig. 3.33.

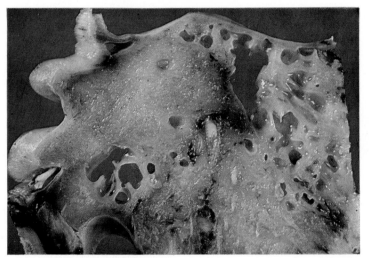

3.35 Photograph of posterior surface of coronal macrosection Fig. 3.33. Reversed photographically.

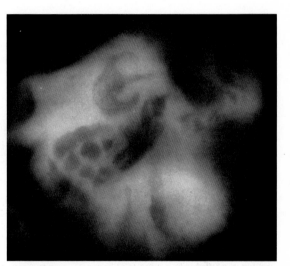

3.36 Tomograph corresponding to Fig. 3.35.

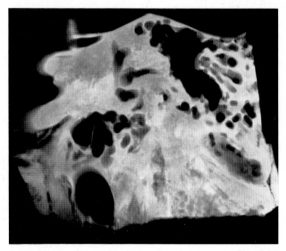

3.37 Microradiograph of macrosection seen in Fig. 3.33 and 3.35.

Coronal Sections

Figures 3.38–3.43 show the structures in a 2 mm thick coronal section of a left adult temporal bone immediately posterior to Figs. 3.32–3.37.
Mastoid air cells extend from the mastoid antrum.

The loop of the posterior semicircular canal lies in the petrosa. The facial nerve descends toward the stylo-mastoid foramen, and the jugular fossa appears at the inferior margin of the section.

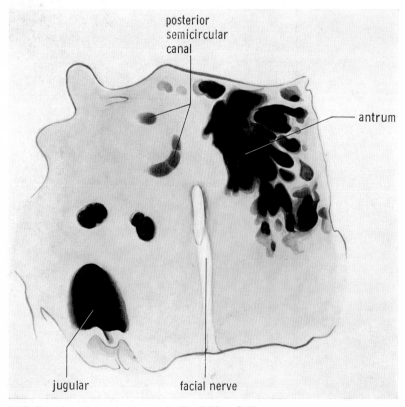

3.38 Drawing of structures seen in Fig. 3.39 to 3.43.

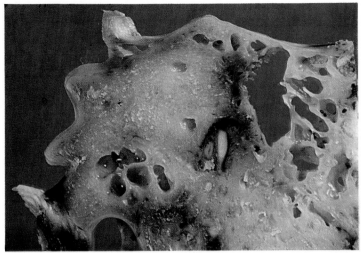

3.39 Photograph of anterior surface of the coronal macrosection immediately posterior to Fig. 3.35.

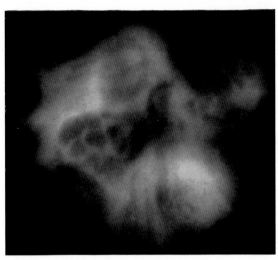

3.40 Tomograph corresponding to Fig. 3.39.

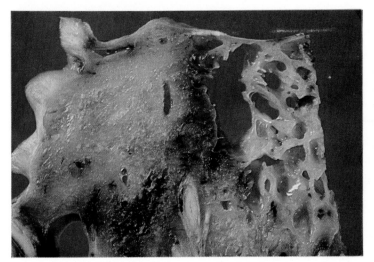

3.41 Photograph of posterior surface of coronal macrosection Fig. 3.39. Reversed photographically.

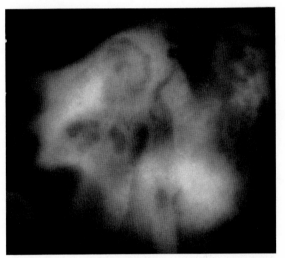

3.42 Tomograph corresponding to Fig. 3.41.

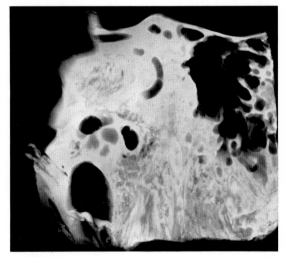

3.43 Microradiograph of macrosection seen in Fig. 3.39 and 3.41.

Chapter 4　Semiaxial Projection of the Petrous Pyramid and Semiaxial Sections

The main purpose of the semiaxial projection is to study the medial or labyrinthine wall of the middle ear cavity. This projection is mandatory for the evaluation of the oval window, the promontory, the horizontal semicircular canal, and the horizontal segment of the facial nerve canal. The semiaxial projection is also satisfactory for the study of the lumen of the middle ear cavity, the ossicles, the floor of the hypotympanum, and the lateral epitympanic wall. We use this projection in the evaluation of cases of otosclerosis, cholesteatoma, facial paralysis and glomus tumor.

The semiaxial projection is obtained by rotating the head of the supine patient 20° toward the side being examined. The medial or labyrinthine wall of the middle ear cavity forms an angle, open posteriorly, of 15° to 25° with the sagittal plane of the skull. By rotating the

skull 20° the medial wall becomes perpendicular to the plane of the film and to the plane of section. We use a plastic box to fix the head of the patient for the coronal and semiaxial projections. For the semiaxial projection, we simply place a 20° wedge under the appropriate side of the box. This allows us to reproduce this view with ease and accuracy if it should be necessary later on (Fig. 4.1).

In this atlas the isolated temporal bone was positioned as for coronal sectioning, and the apex of the pyramid then elevated 20°.

Nine consecutive sections, each 2 mm thick, of a right temporal bone are presented. The photographs of the posterior aspect of each section have been reversed to facilitate comparison with the corresponding tomographs and microradiographs which are included.

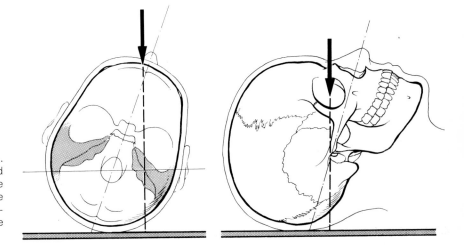

4.1 Semiaxial projection, head position. The sagittal plane of the skull is rotated 20° toward the side to be examined. The tragus canthus line is perpendicular to the film plane. The arrows indicate the position of the centering point on the surface of the head.

Semiaxial Sections

Figures 4.2–4.7 show the structures in a 2 mm thick, semiaxial section of a right adult temporal bone.

The anterior aspect of the first tissue section passes through the eustachian tube portion of the middle ear just anterior to the cochlea and geniculate ganglion.

The canal of the tensor tympani muscle projects from the medial wall of the anterior portion of the middle ear.

On the posterior surface of the section, the geniculate ganglion appears medial to the tensor tympani muscle and above the cochlea (Fig. 4.5 and 4.6). The carotid artery lies underneath the cochlea. The porus of the internal auditory canal notches the medial surface of the petrous pyramid.

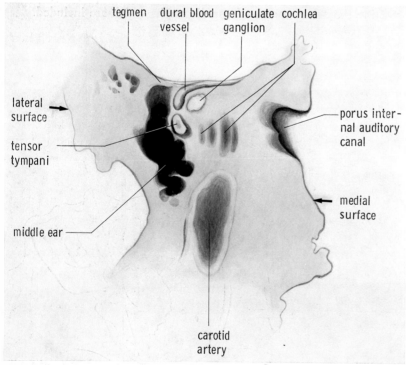

4.2 Drawing of structures seen in Fig. 4.3 to 4.7.

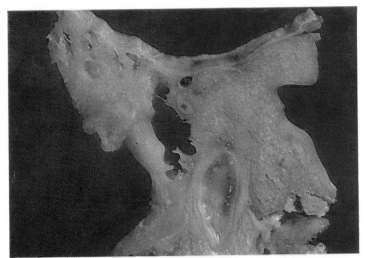

4.3 Photograph of anterior surface of a semiaxial macrosection at the level of the eustachian tube portion of the middle ear.

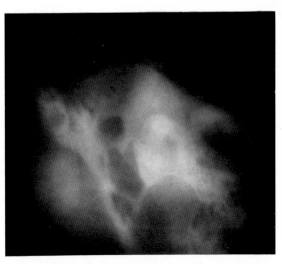

4.4 Tomograph corresponding to Fig. 4.3.

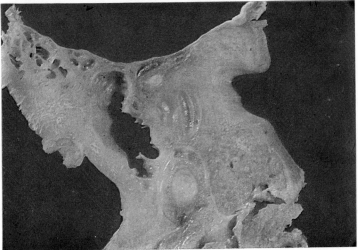

4.5 Photograph of posterior surface of semiaxial macrosection Fig. 4.3. Reversed photographically.

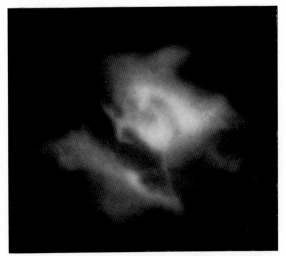

4.6 Tomograph corresponding to Fig. 4.5.

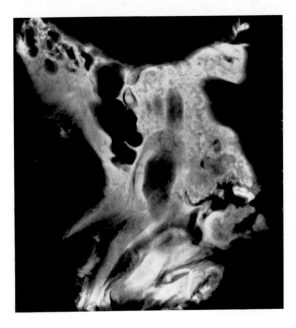

4.7 Microradiograph of macrosection seen in Fig. 4.3 and 4.5.

Semiaxial Sections

Figures 4.8–4.13 show the structures contained in a 2 mm thick, semiaxial section of a right adult temporal bone immediately posterior to Fig. 4.2–4.7.

The section passes through the most anterior portion of the external auditory canal, the anterior portion of the tympanic membrane, the cochlea, and the internal auditory canal. The section exposes the epi-, meso-, and hypotympanums. The tensor tympani muscle projects from the medial wall of the middle ear.

Above the cochlea, the facial nerve bifurcates from the geniculate ganglion into its petrous and tympanic segments.

Portions of three coils of the cochlea lie lateral to the internal auditory canal.

The tomographs show only the contour of the lumen of the spiral canal of the cochlea and the bony septa between the coils, since the spongy modiolus and the spiral lamina are radiolucent at the voltage required to tomograph undecalcified bones.

The carotid artery appears inferior to the cochlea.

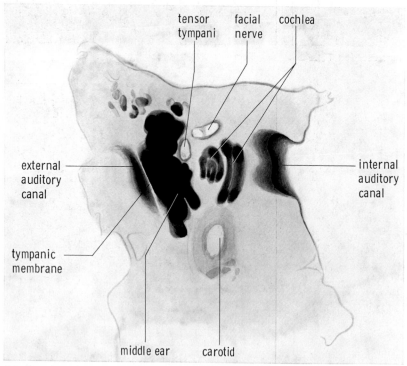

4.8 Drawing of structures seen in Fig. 4.9 to 4.13.

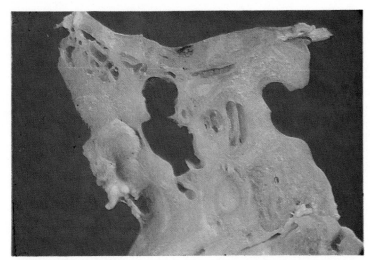

4.9 Photograph of anterior surface of the semiaxial macrosection immediately posterior to Fig. 4.5.

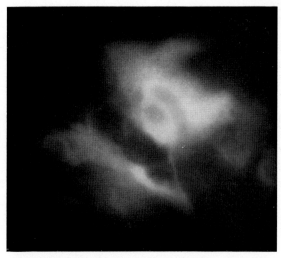

4.10 Tomograph corresponding to Fig. 4.9.

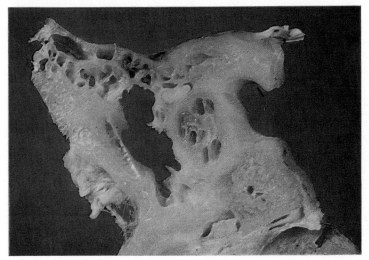

4.11 Photograph of posterior surface of semiaxial macrosection Fig. 4.9. Reversed photographically.

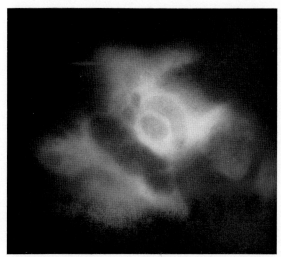

4.12 Tomograph corresponding to Fig. 4.11.

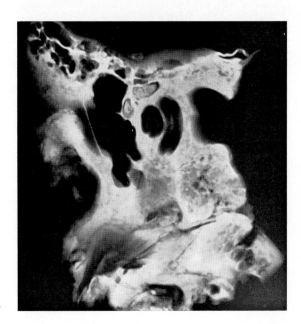

4.13 Microradiograph of macrosection seen in Fig. 4.9 and 4.11.

Semiaxial Sections

Figures 4.14–4.19 show the structures contained in a 2 mm thick semiaxial section of a right adult temporal bone immediately posterior to Fig. 4.8–4.13.

The section exposes a portion of the external auditory canal and an anterior strip of the tympanic membrane.

The head and part of the neck of the malleus lie in the epitympanum. The inferior and anterior margin of the lateral epitympanic wall is in close relation to the malleus neck.

The tensor tympani tendon lies on the medial wall of the middle ear below the horizontal portion of the facial nerve.

The proximal or petrous portion of the facial nerve stretches medially into the lumen of the internal auditory canal above the crista falciformis.

The cochlear nerve passes into the base of the modiolus below the crista faliciformis. Portions of the middle and basal coils of the cochlea lie medial to the fundus of the internal auditory canal.

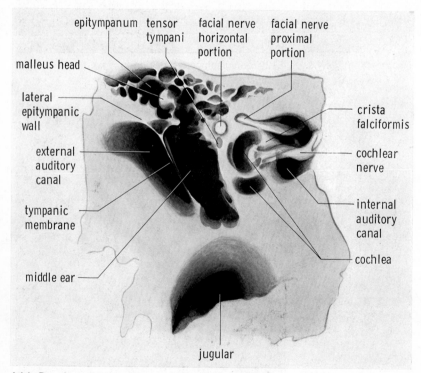

4.14 Drawing of structures seen in Fig. 4.15 to 4.19.

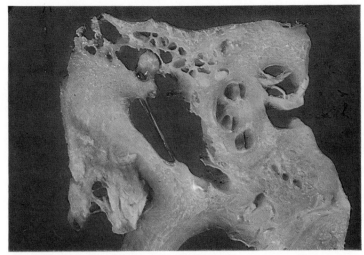

4.15 Photograph of anterior surface of the semiaxial macrosection immediately posterior to Fig. 4.11.

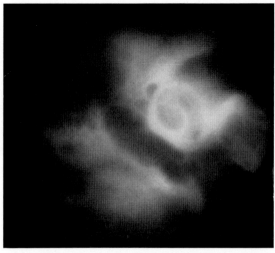

4.16 Tomograph corresponding to Fig. 4.15.

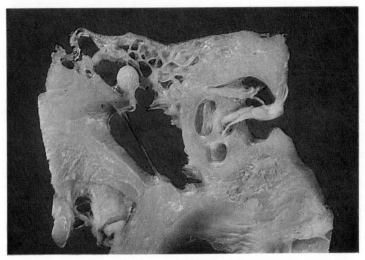

4.17 Photograph of posterior surface of semiaxial macrosection Fig. 4.15. Reversed photographically.

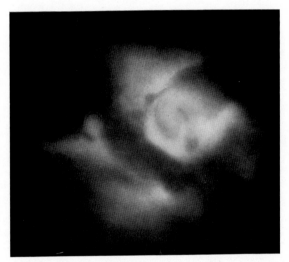

4.18 Tomograph corresponding to Fig. 4.17.

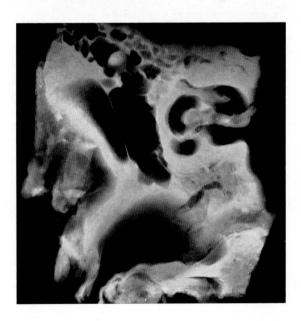

4.19 Microradiograph of macrosection seen in Fig. 4.15 and 4.17

Semiaxial Sections

Figures 4.20–4.25 show the structures contained in a 2 mm thick semiaxial section of a right adult temporal bone immediately posterior to Fig. 4.14–4.19.

The tympanic membrane and malleus handle separate the external canal from the middle ear.

The superior wall of the external auditory canal joins the inferior margin of the lateral attic wall in a sharp projection just above the short process of the malleus. In the epitympanum the body of the incus protrudes lateral from the head of the malleus.

The tendon of the tensor tympani crosses the middle ear from the cochleariform process to the malleus. The horizontal portion of the facial nerve is closely related to the cochleariform process.

The promontory of the basal turn of the cochlea forms the medial wall of the tympanic cavity.

The superior and inferior vestibular nerves flare at the vestibular areas in the fundus of the internal auditory canal (Fig. 4.23). The crista falciformis divides the two branches of the vestibular nerve.

Inferior, a thin wall separates the hypotympanum from the dome of the jugular fossa.

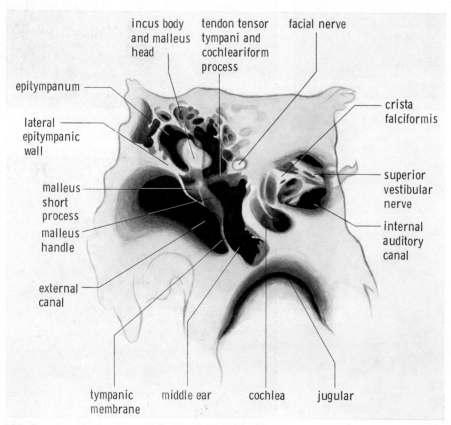

4.20 Drawing of structures seen in Fig. 4.21 to 4.25.

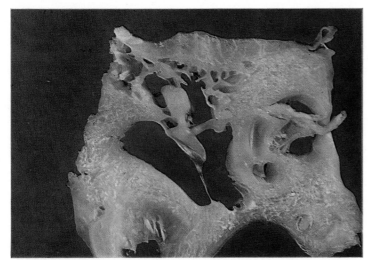

4.21 Photograph of anterior surface of the semiaxial macrosection imme-diately posterior to Fig. 4.17.

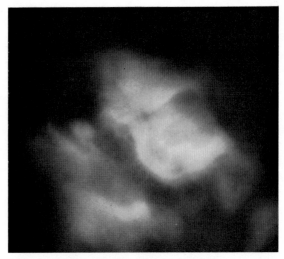

4.22 Tomograph corresponding to Fig. 4.21.

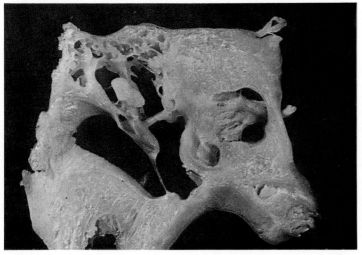

4.23 Photograph of posterior surface of semiaxial macrosection Fig. 4.21. Reversed photographically.

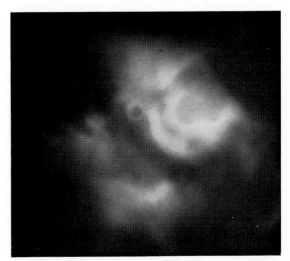

4.24 Tomograph corresponding to Fig. 4.23.

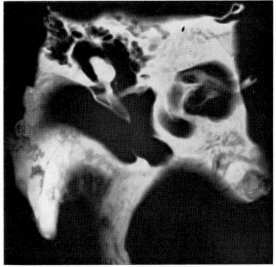

4.25 Microradiograph of macrosection seen in Fig. 4.21 and 4.23.

Semiaxial Sections

Figures 4.26–4.31 show the structures contained in a 2 mm thick semiaxial section of a right adult temporal bone immediately adjacent to Fig. 4.20–4.25.

A strip of the tympanic membrane extends from the inferior margin of the lateral epitympanic wall to the anulus tympanicus inferior. The body of the incus lies in the epitympanum. The long process of the incus extends to articulate with the head of the stapes.

The facial nerve lies in the medial wall of the middle ear below the prominence of the horizontal semicircular canal.

The anterior portion of the stapes footplate closes the oval window. The anterior crus is attached to the footplate.

In the lumen of the promontory, the lamina spiralis separates the scala tympani from the scala vestibuli. The scala vestibuli opens into the vestibule above the scala tympani.

The ampullated ends of the superior and horizontal semicircular canals open into the vestibule. Segments of the membranous semicircular canals, the anterior portion of the utricle, the utricular macula, and the saccule occupy the lumen of the vestibule and bony canals (Fig. 4.29 and 4.31).

Only the fundus of the internal auditory canal remains on the anterior surface of the tissue section (Fig. 4.27).

The distal portion of the cochlear aqueduct opens into the neural portion of the jugular fossa (Fig. 4.31). A thin bony plate separates the jugular dome from the hypotympanum.

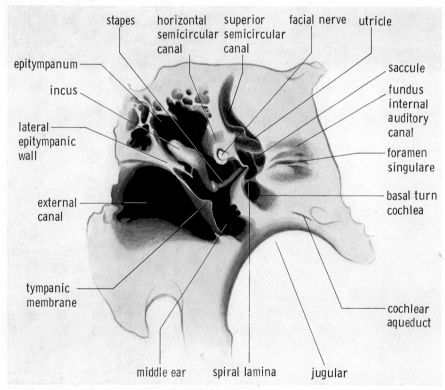

4,26 Drawing of structures seen in Fig. 4.27 to 4.31.

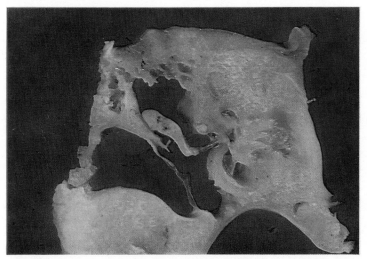

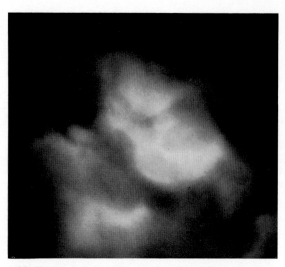

4.27 Photograph of anterior surface of the semiaxial macrosection imme-diately posterior to Fig. 4.23.

4.28 Tomograph corresponding to Fig. 4.27.

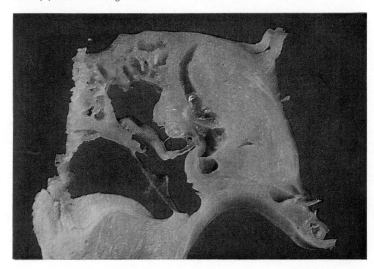

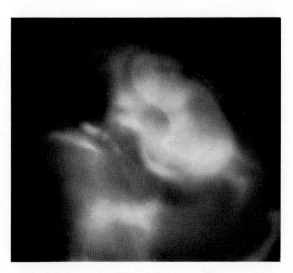

4.29 Photograph of posterior surface of semiaxial macrosection Fig. 4.27. Reversed photographically.

4.30 Tomograph corresponding to Fig. 4.29.

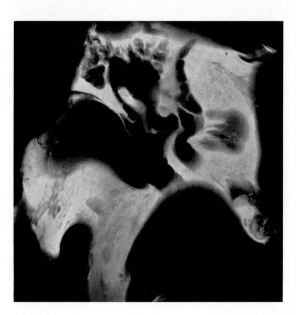

4.31 Microradiograph of macrosection seen in Fig. 4.27 and 4.29.

Semiaxial Sections

Figures 4.32–4.37 demonstrate the structures contained in a 2 mm thick semiaxial section of a right adult temporal bone immediately posterior to Fig. 4.26–4.31.

The section includes the external auditory canal, a thin section of tympanic membrane, the middle ear, and the aditus.

The short process of the incus rests in the fossa incudis above the posterosuperior wall of the external auditory canal.

The horizontal semicircular canal forms the medial boundary of the aditus of the mastoid antrum.

The facial nerve appears under the horizontal semi-circular canal. The posterior half of the stapes footplate closes the oval window, and the posterior crus lies in the oval window niche. In the inferior aspect of the promontory, the round window membrane separates the round window niche from the scala tympani.

The superior semicircular canal arches upwards from the vestibule. The utricle occupies the upper portion of the bony vestibule.

The microradiograph and one tomograph demonstrate the cochlear aqueduct arching within the thickness of the tissue section above the jugular fossa (Fig. 4.34 and 4.37).

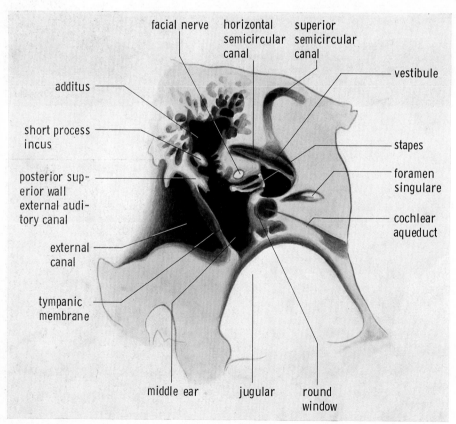

4.32 Drawing of structures seen in Fig. 4.33 to 4.37.

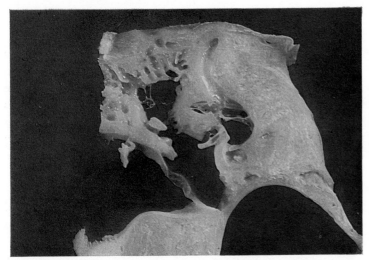

4.33 Photograph of anterior surface of the semiaxial macrosection immediately posterior to Fig. 4.29.

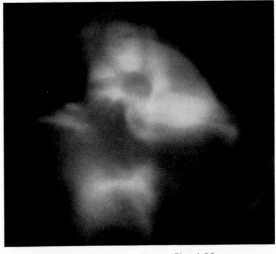

4.34 Tomograph corresponding to Fig. 4.33.

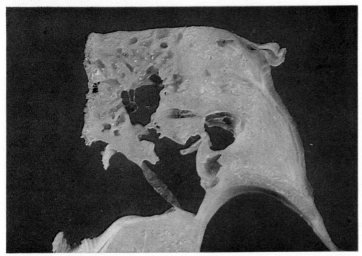

4.35 Photograph of posterior surface of semiaxial macrosection Fig. 4.33. Reversed photographically.

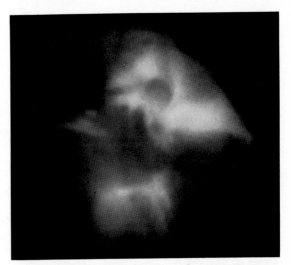

4.36 Tomograph corresponding to Fig. 4.35.

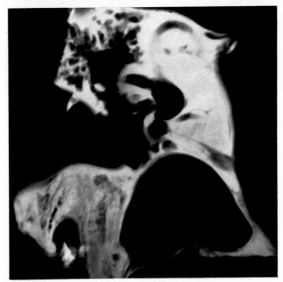

4.37 Microradiograph of macrosection seen in Fig. 4.33 and 4.35.

Semiaxial Sections

Figures 4.38–4.43 demonstrate the structures contained in a 2 mm thick semiaxial section of a right adult temporal bone immediately posterior to Fig. 4.32–4.37.

The section exposes the mastoid antrum with its surrounding air cells, the posterior wall of the external auditory canal, and the posterior part of the tympanic membrane.

The tip of the incus short process lies in the fossa incudis.

The facial nerve and the pyramidal eminence lie in the posterior wall of the middle ear below the antrum.

The dome of the jugular fossa forms the floor of the hypotympanum.

The horizontal semicircular canal projects into the antrum.

The posterior limb of the superior semicircular canal joins the crus commune. On the posterior surface of the section, the ampullated end of the posterior semicircular canal opens into the inferior portion of the vestibule, Fig. 4.41 and 4.42. The posterior margin of the round window lies on the anterior surface of the section opposite the posterior ampulla (Fig. 4.39 and 4.40). Less than 2 mm, the thickness of this section, separates these two structures.

Portions of the membranous labyrinth occupy the lumen of the vestibule.

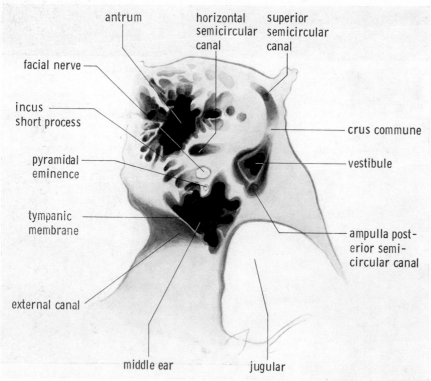

4.38 Drawing of structures seen in Fig. 4.39 to 4.43.

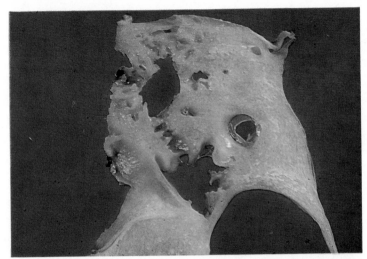

4.39 Photograph of anterior surface of the semiaxial macrosection immediately posterior to Fig. 4.35.

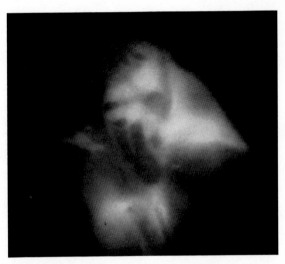

4.40 Tomograph corresponding to Fig. 4.39.

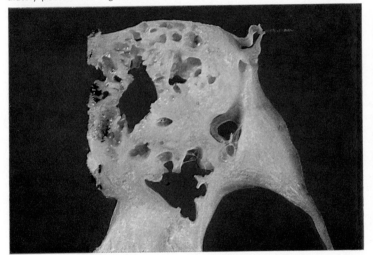

4.41 Photograph of posterior surface of semiaxial macrosection Fig. 4.39.
Reversed photographically.

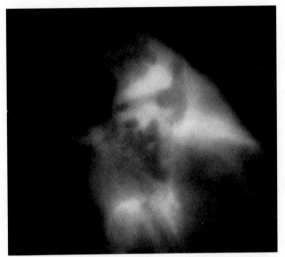

4.42 Tomograph corresponding to Fig. 4.41.

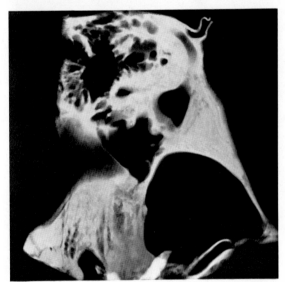

4.43 Microradiograph of macrosection seen in Fig. 4.39
and 4.41.

Semiaxial Sections

Figures 4.44–4.49 reveal the structures contained in a 2 mm thick semiaxial section of a right adult temporal bone immediately posterior to Fig. 4.38–4.43.

The section passes through the antrum and mastoid air cells. The facial nerve turns below the horizontal semicircular canal into the vertical portion. In the tomographs the distal segment of the facial nerve descends to the stylomastoid foramen.

The posterior wall of the middle ear opens into air cells both medial and lateral to the pyramidal process and facial nerve. The air cells medial to the facial nerve form the sinus tympani.

The crus commune, the posterior limb of the horizontal semicircular canal, and the ampulla of the posterior semicircular canal open into the posterior portion of the vestibule.

The jugular fossa lies inferior.

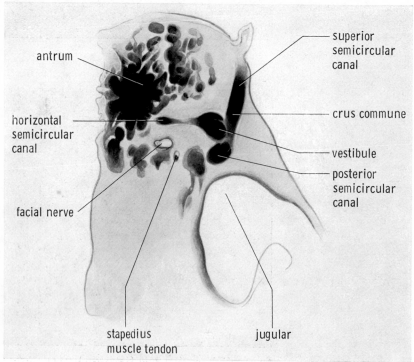

4.44 Drawing of structures seen in Fig. 4.45 to 4.49.

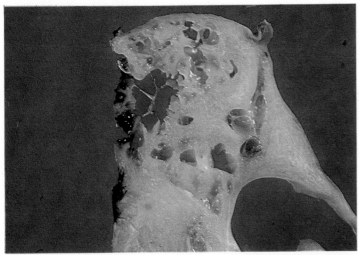

4.45 Photograph of anterior surface of the semiaxial macrosection immediately posterior to Fig. 4.41.

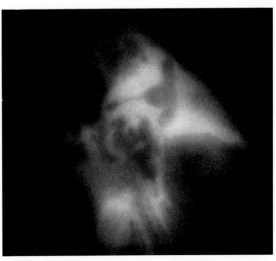

4.46 Tomograph corresponding to Fig. 4.45.

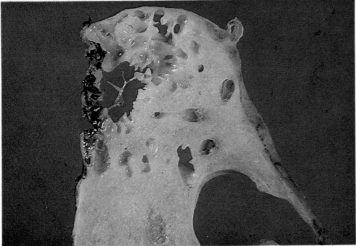

4.47 Photograph of posterior surface of semiaxial macrosection Fig. 4.45. Reversed photographically.

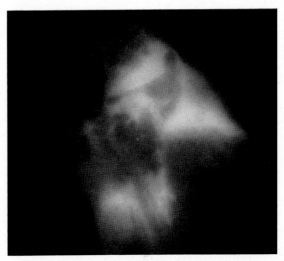

4.48 Tomograph corresponding to Fig. 4.47.

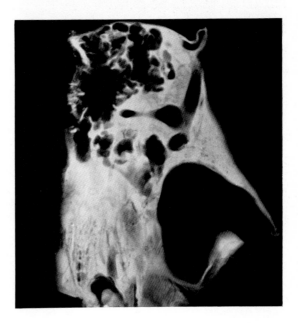

4.49 Microradiograph of macrosection seen in Fig. 4.45 and 4.47.

Semiaxial Sections

Figures 4.50–4.55 depict the structures within a 2 mm thick semiaxial section of a right adult temporal bone immediately posterior to Fig. 4.44–4.49.

The mastoid air cells make up the upper portion of the section. The facial nerve descends toward the stylo- mastoid foramen. The posterior semicircular canal arches above the jugular fossa.

The stapedius muscle lies between the descending portion of the facial nerve and lateral aspect of the jugular fossa.

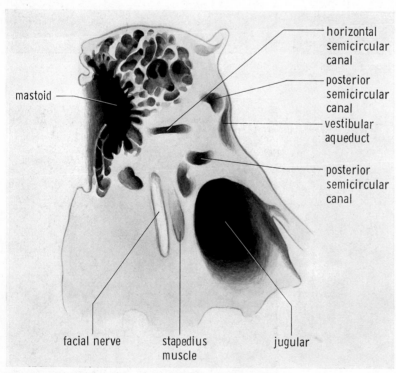

4.50 Drawing of structures seen in Fig. 4.51 to 4.55.

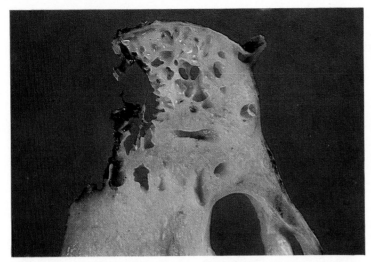

4.51 Photograph of anterior surface of the semiaxial macrosection immediately posterior to Fig. 4.47.

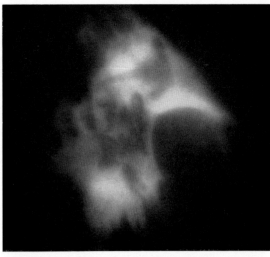

4.52 Tomograph corresponding to Fig. 4.51.

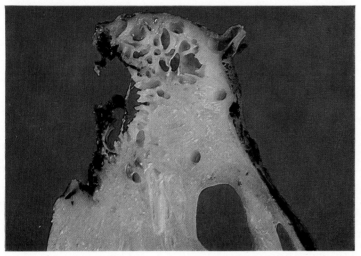

4.53 Photograph of posterior surface of semiaxial macrosection Fig. 4.51. Reversed photographically.

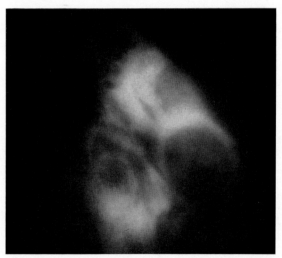

4.54 Tomograph corresponding to Fig. 4.53.

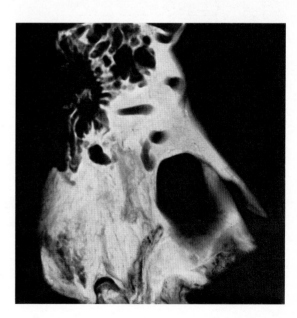

4.55 Microradiograph of macrosection seen in Fig. 4.51 and 4.53.

Chapter 5   Axial Projection of the Petrous Pyramid and Axial Sections

The axial projection is used by European radiologists to study the cochlear capsule. The section or sections through the long axis of the modiolus allow good visualization, on end, of several segments of the cochlear coil. We employ this projection in combination with sagittal sections to study the vestibular aqueduct. The increase thickness of the temporal bone in this projection calls for an increase in the amount and penetration of the x-rays, which, in our opinion, is objectionable unless the desired information cannot be obtained from other projections.

The axial projection is obtained with the patient supine and the head rotated, as for the Mayers view, 45° toward the side being examined (Fig. 5.1).
In this atlas the isolated temporal bones were positioned with the posterior surface of the petrous pyramid perpendicular to the plane of the film.
Nine consecutive sections of a left temporal bone are shown, each 2 mm thick. The photographs of the anteromedial aspect of each section have been reversed to facilitate comparison with the corresponding tomograms and microradiographs which are included.

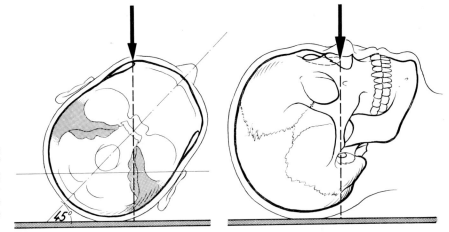

5.1 Axial projection, head position. The sagittal plane of the skull is rotated 45° toward the side to be examined. The long axis of the petrous pyramid is perpendicular to the film plane. The arrows indicate the position of the centering point on the surface of the head.

Axial Sections

The first illustrations (Fig. 5.2–5.7) show the structures present in a 2 mm thick axial section of a left adult temporal bone at the level of the medial end of the external auditory canal, the posterior portion of the annulus tympanicus, and the mastoid air cells.

The prominence of the horizontal semicircular canal projects into the antrum. The arch of the posterior semicircular canal lies behind and at right angles to the horizontal semicircular canal.

The short process of the incus rests in the fossa incudis above the posterosuperior wall of the external auditory canal.

The facial nerve descends below the horizontal semicircular canal from the pyramidal turn to the stylomastoid foramen.

The chorda tympani leaves the facial nerve at the level of the floor of the external auditory canal.

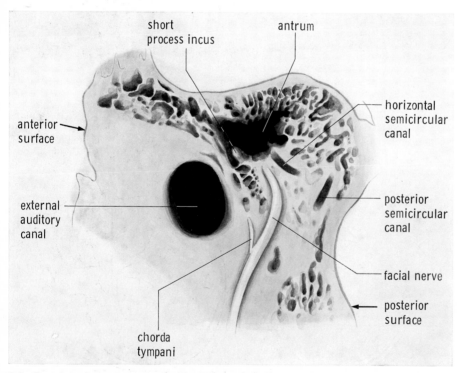

5.2   Drawing of structures seen in Fig. 5.3 to 5.7.

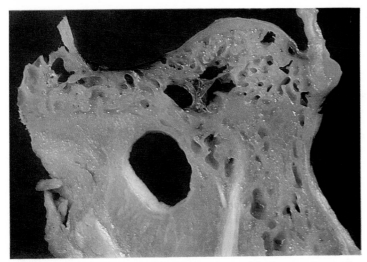

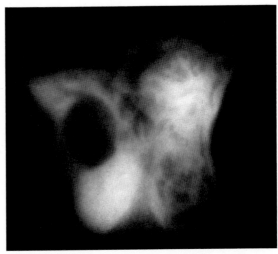

5.3 Photograph of posterolateral surface of an axial macrosection at the level of the medial end of the external auditory canal.

5.4 Tomograph corresponding to Fig. 5.3.

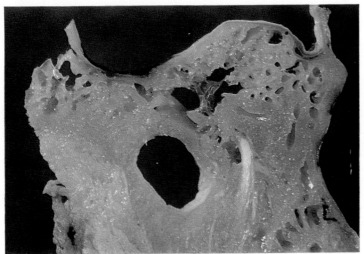

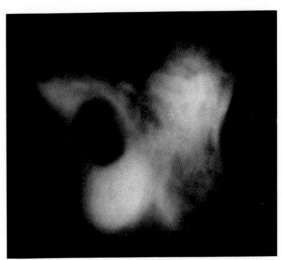

5.5 Photograph of anteromedial surface of axial macrosection Fig. 5.3. Reversed photographically.

5.6 Tomograph corresponding to Fig. 5.5.

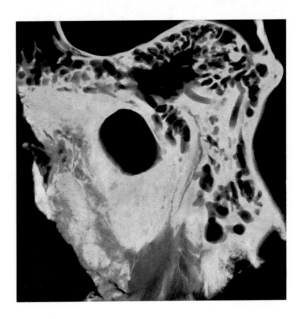

5.7 Microradiograph of macrosection seen in Fig. 5.3 and 5.5.

Axial Sections

Figures 5.8–5.13 show the structures contained in a 2 mm thick axial section of a left adult temporal bone immediately anteromedial to Fig. 5.2–5.7.

The section crosses the posterosuperior wall of the external auditory canal and passes through the posterior portion of the annular ligament.

The epitympanum contains a section of the body of the incus.

The tegmen tympani and the prominence of the horizontal semicircular canal bound the epitympanum.

The posterior semicircular canal arches behind the horizontal semicircular canal.

The facial nerve approaches the pyramidal turn below the horizontal semicircular canal.

The space between the posterior wall of the external canal and the facial nerve is the facial recess. Some otologists use this area as a surgical approach to the middle ear.

On the posterior surface of the section the endolymphatic sac passes into the vestibular aqueduct.

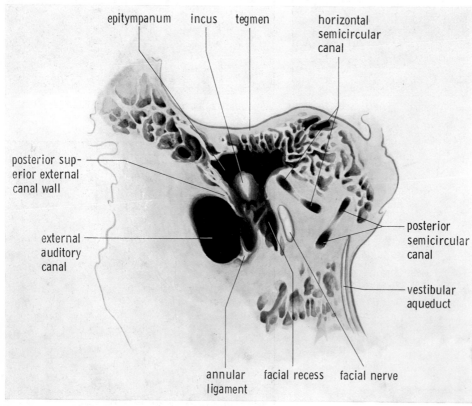

5.8 Drawing of structures seen in Fig. 5.9 to 5.13.

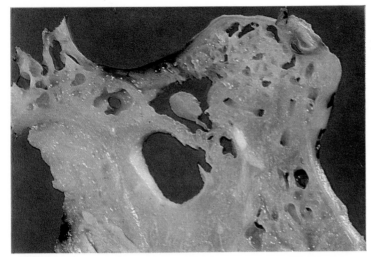

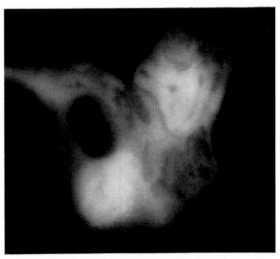

5.9 Photograph of posterolateral surface of the axial macrosection immediately anteromedial to Fig. 5.5.

5.10 Tomograph corresponding to Fig. 5.9.

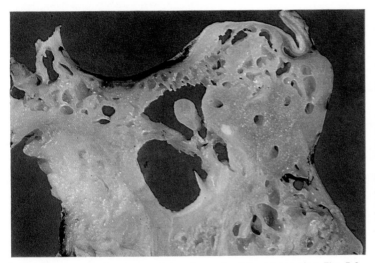

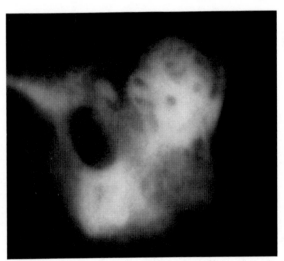

5.11 Photograph of anteromedial surface of axial macrosection Fig. 5.9. Reversed photographically.

5.12 Tomograph corresponding to Fig. 5.11.

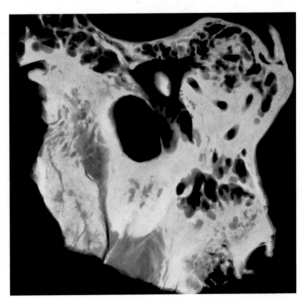

5.13 Microradiograph of macrosection seen in Fig. 5.9 and 5.11.

Axial Sections

Figures 5.14–5.19 reveal the structures contained in a 2 mm thick axial section of a left adult temporal bone immediately anteromedial to Fig. 5.8–5.13.

A strip of the tympanic membrane and a section of the chorda tympani, parallel to the membrane, separate the external canal from the middle ear cavity.

The malleus head and the body of the incus occupy the epitympanum. The long process of the incus extends into the tympanic cavity.

The anterior tympanic spine projects just above the short process of the malleus.

The facial nerve is beneath the horizontal semicircular canal.

Cross sections of the superior, horizontal, and posterior semicircular canals are present posterior.

The vestibular aqueduct extends upwards from the posterior surface of the section towards the upper limb of the posterior semicircular canal.

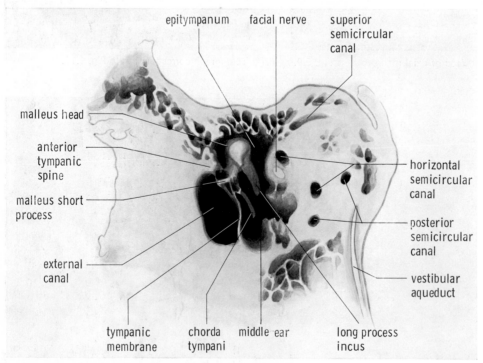

5.14 Drawing of structures seen in Fig. 5.15 to 5.19.

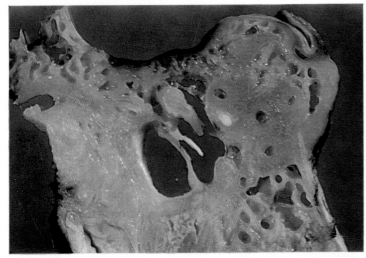

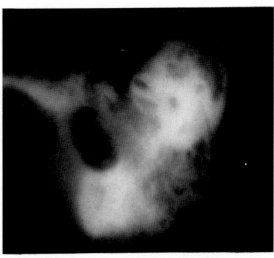

5.15 Photograph of posterolateral surface of the axial macrosection immediately anteromedial to Fig. 5.11.

5.16 Tomograph corresponding to Fig. 5.15.

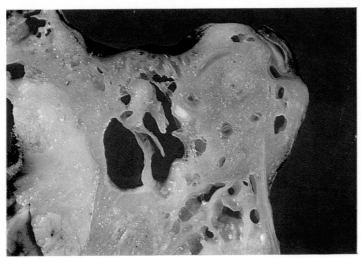

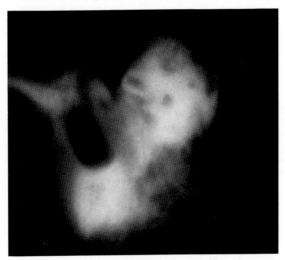

5.17 Photograph of anteromedial surface of axial macrosection Fig. 5.15. Reversed photographically.

5.18 Tomograph corresponding to Fig. 5.17.

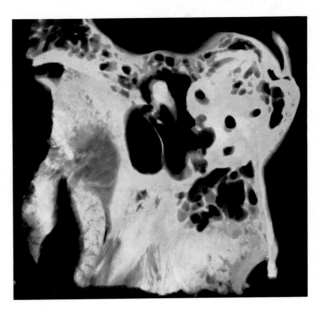

5.19 Microradiograph of macrosection seen in Fig. 5.15 and 5.17.

Axial Sections

Figures 5.20–5.25 show the structures contained in a 2 mm thick axial section of a left adult temporal bone immediately anteromedial to Fig. 5.14–5.19.

The tympanic membrane and the malleus handle demarcate the external canal from the middle ear.

A portion of the tensor tympani tendon is attached to the malleus neck and divides the epitympanum from the mesotympanum. The facial nerve lies on the medial wall of the middle ear opposite the tensor tympani tendon.

In the tomograph, the shadow of the ossicles persists. (Fig. 5.22).

The superior semicircular canal arches through the thickness of the section from the ampullated end to the crus commune. The posterior semicircular canal joins the superior at the crus commune.

The ampullated end of the posterior semicircular canal opens into the inferior portion of the vestibule.

The ampullated and nonampullated limbs of the horizontal semicircular canal enter the upper portion of the vestibule.

The utricle and portions of the membranous semicircular canals occupy their respective bony compartments.

The posterior half of the stapes footplate and a portion of the stapes superstructure lie in the oval window.

The section exposes the promontory, the round window, and the round window niche.

The beginning of the scala vestibuli and scala tympani appears in this segment of the promontory.

The vestibular aqueduct passes upwards toward the crus commune. The jugular fossa lies inferior.

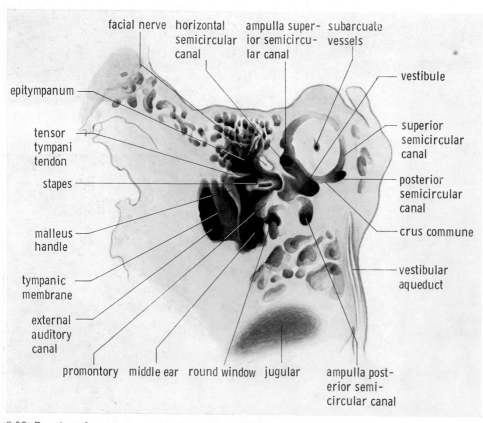

5.20 Drawing of structures seen in Fig. 5.21 to 5.25.

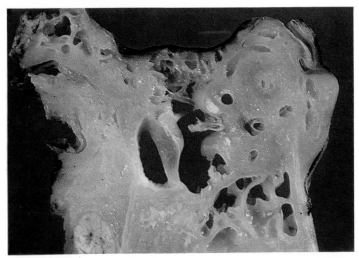

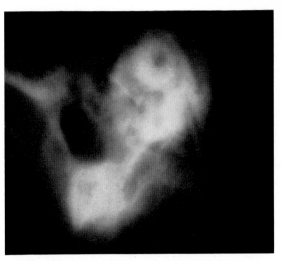

5.21 Photograph of posterolateral surface of the axial macrosection immediately anteromedial to Fig. 5.17.

5.22 Tomograph corresponding to Fig. 5.21.

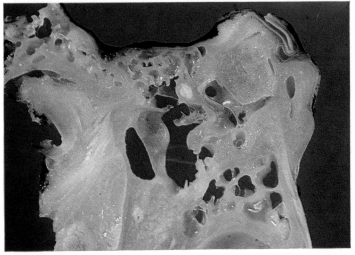

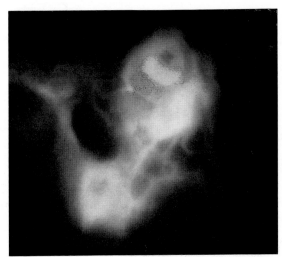

5.23 Photograph of anteromedial surface of axial macrosection Fig. 5.21. Reversed photographically.

5.24 Tomograph corresponding to Fig. 5.23.

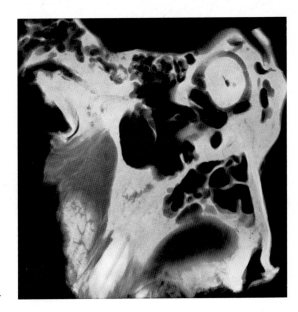

5.25 Microradiograph of macrosection seen in Fig. 5.21 and 5.23.

Axial Sections

Figures 5.26–5.31 reveal the structures contained in a 2 mm thick axial section of a left adult temporal bone immediately anteromedial to Fig. 5.20–5.25.

A small portion of the anterior external auditory canal wall and tympanic membrane remain anterior to the middle ear.

The facial nerve and cochleariform process lie above the anterior part of the oval window. A portion of the anterior crus and a segment of the stapes footplate lie in the oval window above the promontory.

The utricle with the macula fills the upper portion of the vestibule. The superior vestibular nerve passes to the utricular macula. The ampulla of the posterior semicircular canal enters the vestibule inferior.

The scala vestibuli begins at the inferior portion of the vestibule. The scala tympani and round window lie below the scala vestibuli.

Hypotympanic air cells separate the jugular fossa from the floor of the middle ear.

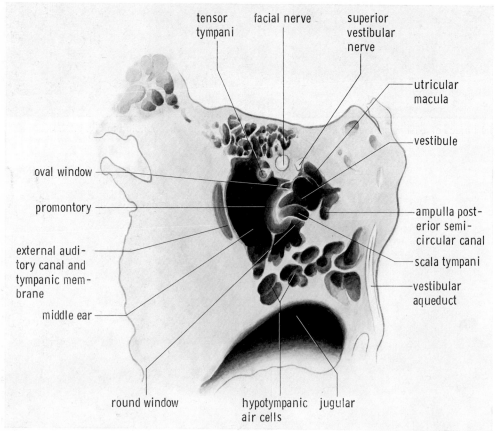

5.26 Drawing of structures seen in Fig. 5.27 to 5.31.

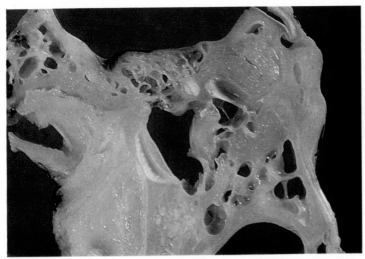

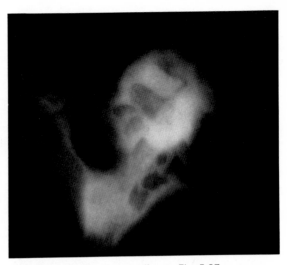

5.27 Photograph of posterolateral surface of the axial macrosection immediately anteromedial to Fig. 5.23.

5.28 Tomograph corresponding to Fig. 5.27.

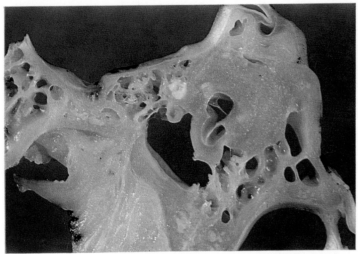

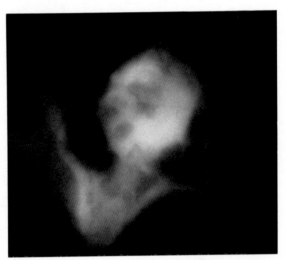

5.29 Photograph of anteromedial surface of axial macrosection Fig. 5.27. Reversed photographically.

5.30 Tomograph corresponding to Fig. 5.29.

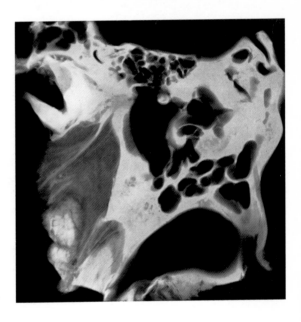

5.31 Microradiograph of macrosection seen in Fig. 5.27 and 5.29.

Axial Sections

Figures 5.32–5.37 expose the structures in a 2 mm thick axial section of a left adult temporal bone immediately anteromedial to Fig. 5.26–5.31.

The section passes through the anterior portion of the middle ear. The canal of the tensor tympani muscle lies just underneath the geniculate ganglion of the facial nerve. There is vacuolization of the geniculate ganglion. The basal turn of the cochlea lies inferior to the spherical recess and saccular macula which form the most anterior medial portion of the vestibule (Fig. 5.33).

The fundus of the internal auditory canal lies on the opposite surface of the section (Fig. 5.35). The inferior vestibular nerve passes to the macula of the saccule within the thickness of the section.

The cochlear aqueduct exits from the scala tympani. A small portion of the middle cochlear coil is present anterior to the fundus of the internal auditory canal.

The jugular fossa bounds the section inferiorly.

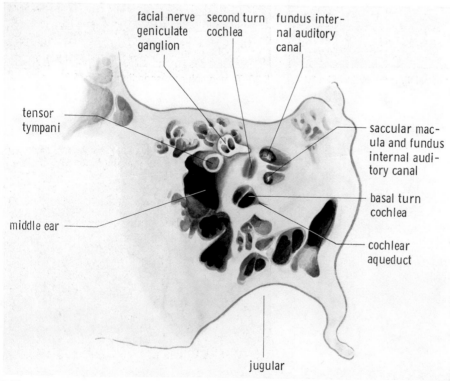

5.32 Drawing of structures seen in Fig. 5.33 to 5.37.

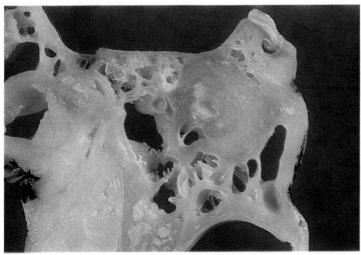

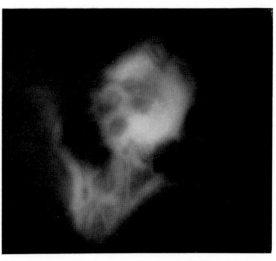

5.33 Photograph of posterolateral surface of the axial macrosection immediately anteromedial to Fig. 5.29.

5.34 Tomograph corresponding to Fig. 5.33.

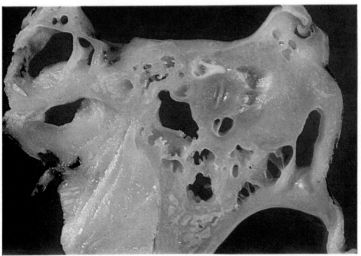

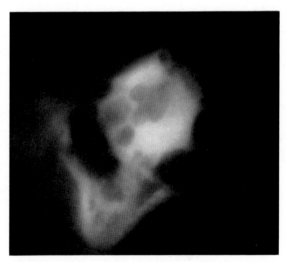

5 35 Photograph of anteromedial surface of axial macrosection Fig. 5.35. Reversed photographically.

5.36 Tomograph corresponding to Fig. 5.35.

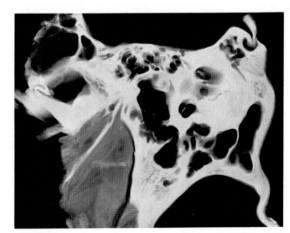

5.37 Microradiograph of macrosection seen in Fig. 5.33 and 5.35.

Axial Sections

Figures 5.38–5.43 show the structures in a 2 mm thick axial section of a left adult temporal bone immediately anteromedial to Fig. 5.32–5.37.

The section passes through the eustachian tube portion of the middle ear. The tensor tympani occupies the superior portion of the lumen of the middle ear. The facial nerve arches from the geniculate ganglion to the internal auditory canal above the cochlea.

The section bisects the modiolus and reveals portions of three cochlear coils.

Petrous air cells surround the otic capsule.

Anterior to the cochlea, the lateral wall of the carotid canal forms part of the medial wall of the middle ear. The jugular fossa forms the posteroinferior margin of the section.

Above the jugular, the cochlear aqueduct lies within the thickness of the section (Fig. 5.43).

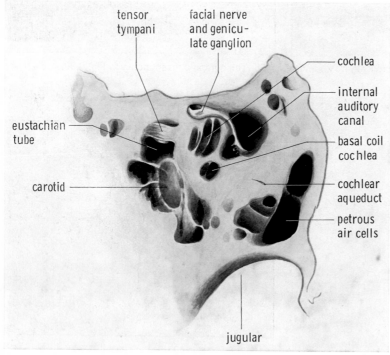

5.38 Drawing of structures seen in Fig. 5.39 to 5.43.

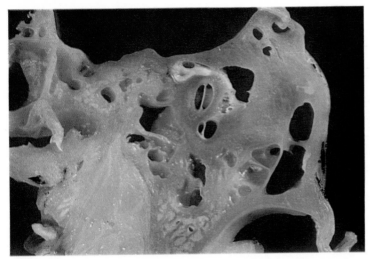

5.39 Photograph of posterolateral surface of the axial macrosection immediately anteromedial to Fig. 5.35.

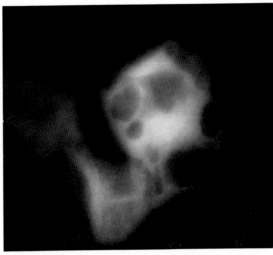

5.40 Tomograph corresponding to Fig. 5.39.

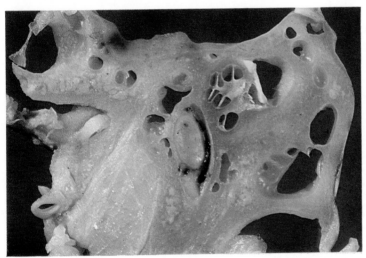

5.41 Photograph of anteromedial surface of axial macrosection Fig. 5.39. Reversed photographically.

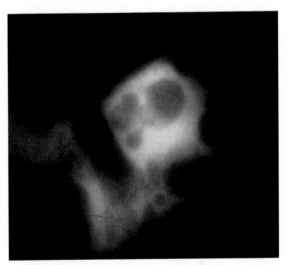

5.42 Tomograph corresponding to Fig. 5.41.

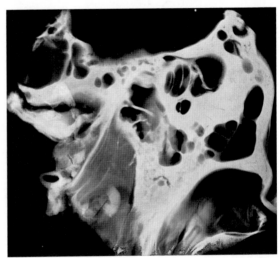

5.43 Microradiograph of macrosection seen in Fig. 5.39 and 5.41.

Axial Sections

Figures 5.44–5.49 show the structures in a 2 mm thick axial section of a left adult temporal bone immediately anteromedial to Fig. 5.38–5.43.

The eustachian portion of the middle ear and the tensor tympani canal abut the carotid artery canal.

The cochlear nerve passes from the internal auditory canal into the base of the modiolus. Parts of three cochlear coils appear in this section. The cochlear aqueduct appears again in the microradiograph (Fig. 5. 49).

The jugular fossa lies inferior.

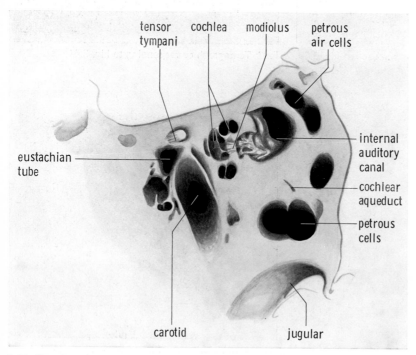

5.44 Drawing of structures seen in Fig. 5.45 to 5.49.

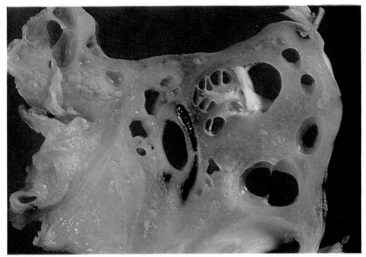

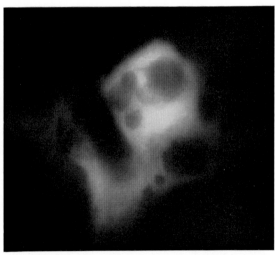

5.45 Photograph of posterolateral surface of the axial macrosection imme-diately anteromedial to Fig. 5.41.

5.46 Tomograph corresponding to Fig. 5.45.

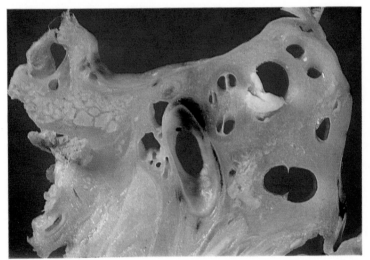

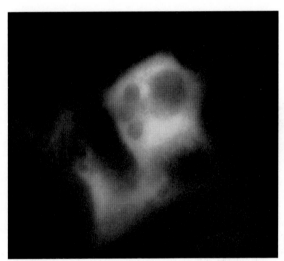

5.47 Photograph of anteromedial surface of axial macrosection Fig. 5.45. Reversed photographically.

5.48 Tomograph corresponding to Fig. 5.47.

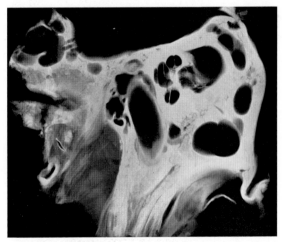

5.49 Microradiograph of macrosection seen in Fig. 5.45 and 5.47.

Axial Sections

Figures 5.50–5.55 expose the structures in a 2 mm thick axial section of a left adult temporal bone immediately anteromedial to Fig. 5.44–5.49.

The section exposes the middle ear portion of the eustachian tube. The tensor tympani canal lies just below the superior surface of the section. The carotid artery remains in close relation to the cochlea. The basal turn of the cochlea is anterior to the internal auditory meatus which contains segments of the facial and acoustic nerves. The cochlear aqueduct descends inferior (Fig. 5.55).

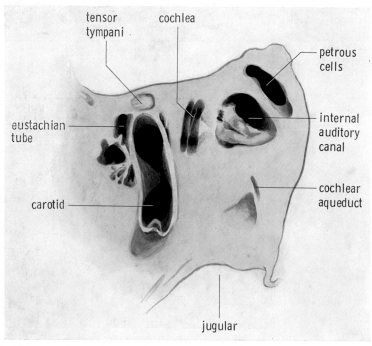

5.50 Drawing of structures seen in Fig. 5.51 to 5.55.

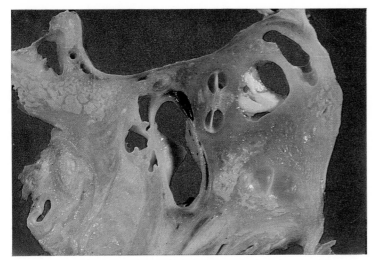

5.51 Photograph of posterolateral surface of the axial macrosection immediately anteromedial to Fig. 5.47.

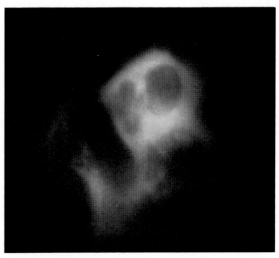

5.52 Tomograph corresponding to Fig. 5.51.

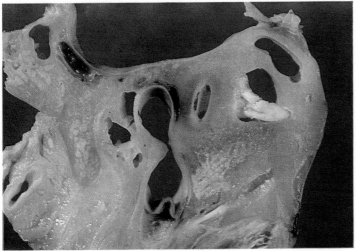

5.53 Photograph of anteromedial surface of axial macrosection Fig. 5.51. Reversed photographically.

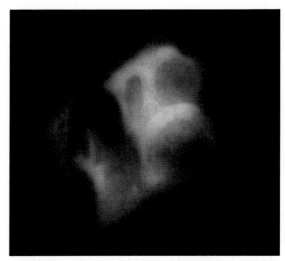

5.54 Tomograph corresponding to Fig. 5.53.

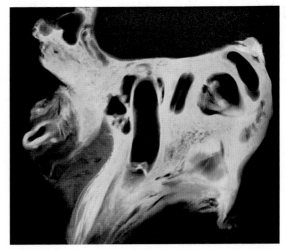

5.55 Microradiograph of macrosection seen in Fig. 5.51 and 5.53.

Chapter 6   Sagittal Projection and Sagittal Sections

The sagittal projection is complementary to the coronal since it shows the anterior to posterior aspects of the structures seen in their lateral to medial relationships in the coronal projection. The sagittal projection is particularly satisfactory for studying the mastoid, external auditory canal, ossicles, vertical portion of the facial nerve canal, semicircular canals, internal auditory canal, and vestibular aqueduct. In addition to being easily obtained and reproduced, this view has the advantage of following the plane of surgical approach. We use the sagittal projection routinely except in the study of the labyrinthine windows and capsule. The patient lies prone on the table, the shoulder of the side

being examined is slightly elevated, and the head rotated until the sagittal plane of the skull becomes parallel to the plane of the film (Fig. 6.1).

In this atlas, the isolated temporal bone was positioned with the mastoid process on the table top and the long axis of the posterior aspect of the petrous pyramid at 135° to the plane of the film.

Nine consecutive tissue sections of the right temporal bone and corresponding tomographs and microradiographs are shown. The photographs of the medial aspect of each section have been reversed in order to facilitate comparison with the tomograms and microradiographs.

6.1   Sagittal projection, head position. The sagittal plane of the skull is parallel to the film plane. The arrows indicate the position of the centering point on the surface of the head.

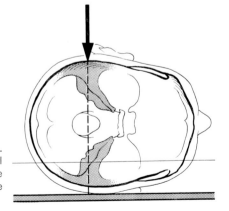
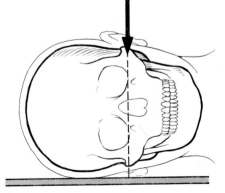

Sagittal Sections

The first sagittal section (Fig. 6.2–6.7), 2 mm thick, of this right adult temporal bone crosses the medial portion of the external auditory canal and the lateral portion of the epitympanum.

A small section of the tympanic membrane is attached to the posterosuperior wall of the external auditory canal

The body of the incus is in the epitympanum and the short process in the fossa incudis.
The tegmen of the middle ear and mastoid forms the upper margin of the tissue section.
Mucosal strands stretch across the mastoid antrum. There are many small air cells in the mastoid.
The vertical portion of the facial nerve descends inferior.

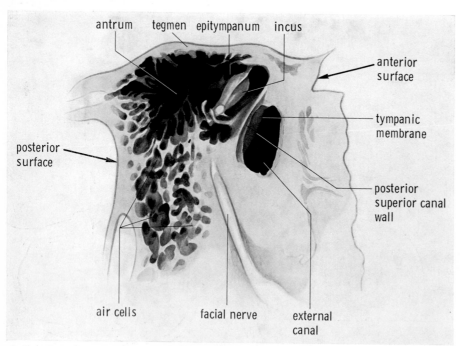

6.2 Drawing of structures seen in Fig. 6.3 to 6.7.

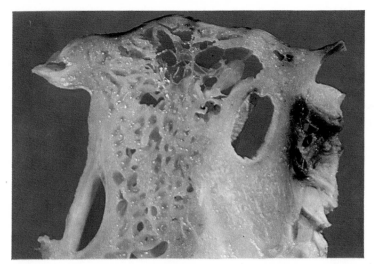

6.3 Photograph of lateral surface of a sagittal macrosection at the level of the lateral portion of the epitympanum.

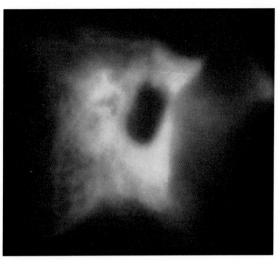

6.4 Tomograph corresponding to Fig. 6.3.

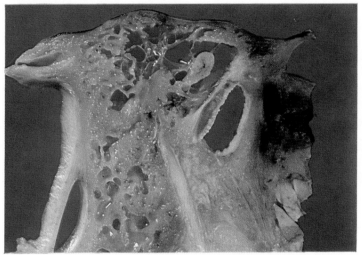

6.5 Photograph of medial surface of sagittal macrosection Fig. 6.3. Reversed photographically.

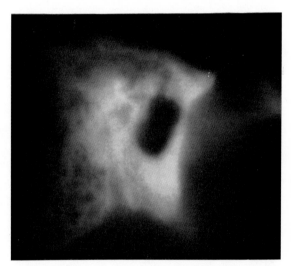

6.6 Tomograph corresponding to Fig. 6.5.

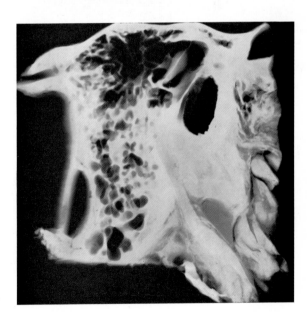

6.7 Microradiograph of macrosection seen in Fig. 6.3 and 6.5.

Sagittal Sections

Figures 6.8–6.13 demonstrate the structures in the 2 mm thick sagittal section of a right adult temporal bone immediately medial to Fig. 6.2–6.7.

A thin strip of the tympanic membrane separates the external auditory canal anterior from the middle ear posterior.

The malleus head and neck occupy the anterior portion of the epitympanum.

The transected incus body articulates with the malleus head.

The short process of the malleus lies in contact with the tympanic membrane. The anterior tympanic spine is just anterior to the malleus short process. A segment of the chorda tympani crosses the middle ear.

The most lateral portions of the horizontal and posterior semicircular canals appear posteriorly.

The facial nerve descends from the pyramidal turn towards the stylomastoid foramen.

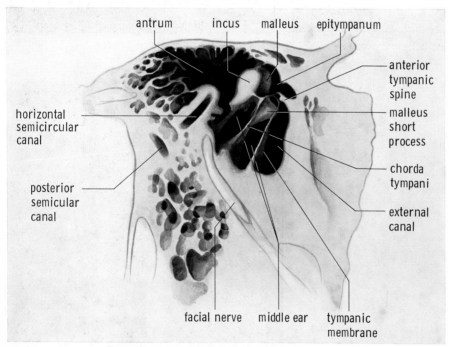

6.8   Drawing of structures seen in Fig. 6.9 to 6.13.

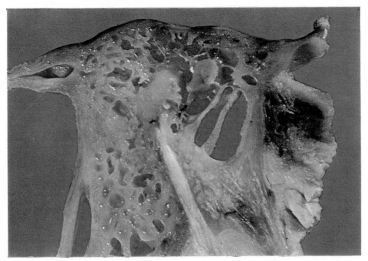

6.9 Photograph of lateral surface of the sagittal macrosection immediately medial to Fig. 6.5.

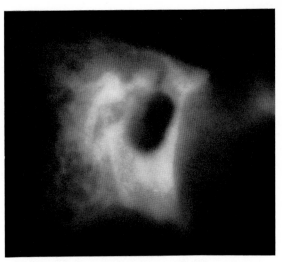

6.10 Tomograph corresponding to Fig. 6.9.

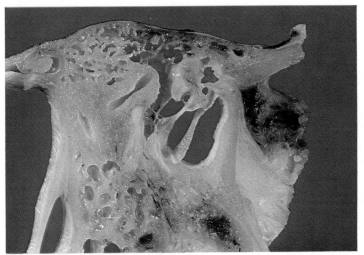

6.11 Photograph of medial surface of sagittal macrosection Fig. 6.9. Reversed photographically.

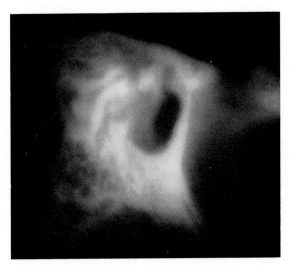

6.12 Tomograph corresponding to Fig. 6.11.

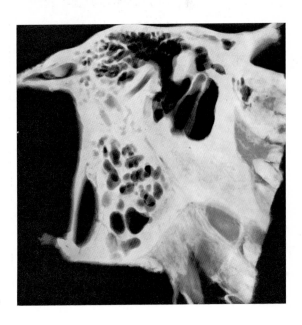

6.13 Microradiograph of macrosection seen in Fig. 6.9 and 6.11.

Sagittal Sections

Figures 6.14–6.19 demonstrate the structures in a 2 mm thick sagittal section of a right adult temporal bone immediately medial to Fig. 6.8–6.13.

A thin strip of tympanic membrane attached to the malleus handle separates the external canal from the middle ear.

The anterior mallear ligament passes into the petrotympanic fissure above the anterior tympanic spine.

The remnant of the body of the incus articulates with the malleus head. The long process of the incus extends to the lenticular process. The horizontal and posterior semicircular canals are in the bone of the petrosa.

A segment of the facial nerve passes below the horizontal semicircular canal.

The pyramidal eminence and stapedius muscle are inferior to the facial nerve.

The endolymphatic sac lies beneath the dura of the posterior surface of the section.

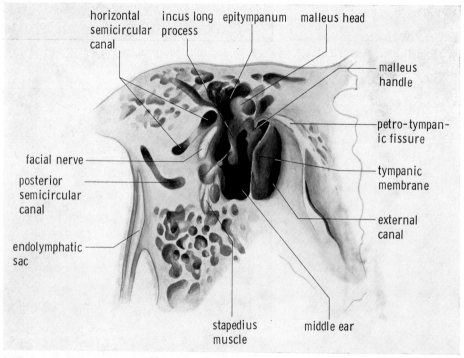

6.14 Drawing of structures seen in Fig. 6.15 to 6.19.

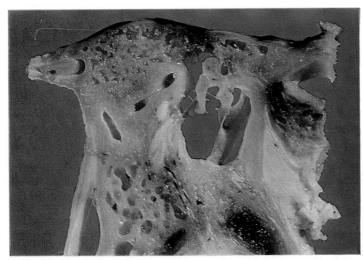

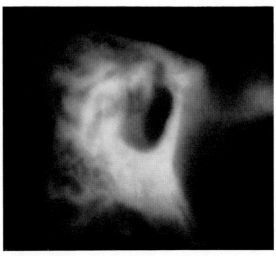

6.15 Photograph of lateral surface of the sagittal macrosection immediately medial to Fig. 6.11.

6.16 Tomograph corresponding to Fig. 6.15.

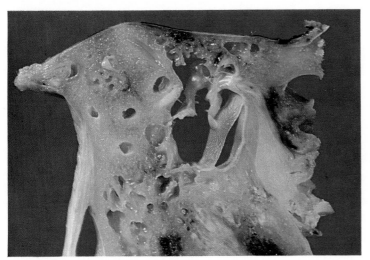

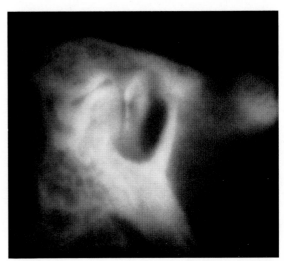

6.17 Photograph of medial surface of sagittal macrosection Fig. 6.15. Reversed photographically.

6.18 Tomograph corresponding to Fig. 6.17.

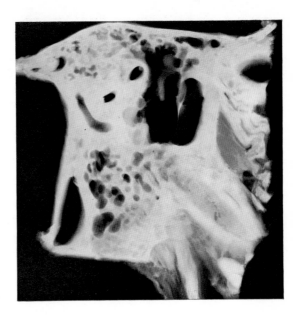

6.19 Microradiograph of macrosection seen in Fig. 6.15 and 6.17.

Sagittal Sections

Figures 6.20–6.25 show the structures in a 2 mm thick sagittal section of a right adult temporal bone immediately medial to Fig. 6.14–6.19.

The section includes the most anterior portion of the external auditory canal, the anterior portion of the tympanic membrane, and a thin section of the cochlear promontory.

The posterior half of the stapes footplate, head, and posterior crus occupy the oval window niche.

The tympanic sinus extends posteriorly from the area between the oval and round windows (Fig. 6.21 and 6.17).

A section of the facial nerve is above the oval window. The cochleariform process and tensor tympani tendon are anterior to the facial nerve.

The three semicircular canals occupy the petrosa posteriorly. Segments of the membranous semicircular canals including their ampullated portions lie in the canal lumina.

The ampullated end of the horizontal semicircular canal opens into the vestibule just below the ampulla of the superior semicircular canal.

The medial surface of the section exposes the most lateral portion of the vestibule, the medial surface of the stapes footplate, and the round window niche and membrane (Fig. 6.23).

The entrance of the endolymphatic sac into the vestibular aqueduct appears on the posterior aspect of the section.

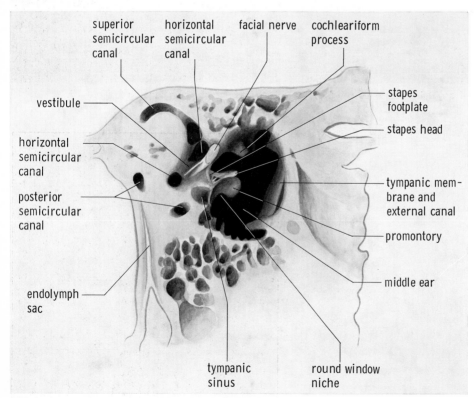

6.20 Drawing of structures seen in Fig. 6.21 to 6.25.

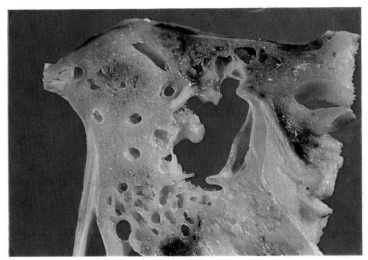

6.21 Photograph of lateral surface of the sagittal macrosection immediately medial to Fig. 6.17.

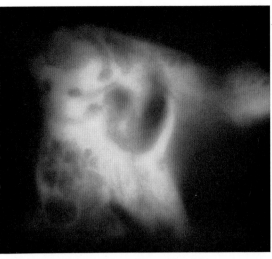

6.22 Tomograph corresponding to Fig. 6.21.

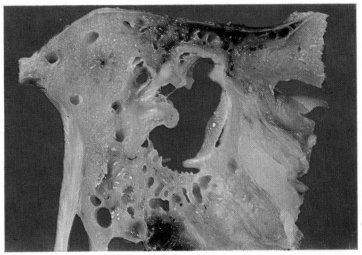

6.23 Photograph of medial surface of sagittal macrosection Fig. 6.21. Reversed photographically.

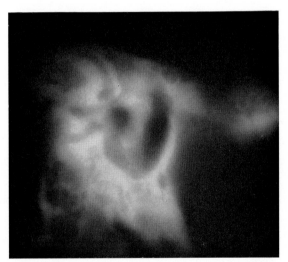

6.24 Tomograph corresponding to Fig. 6.23.

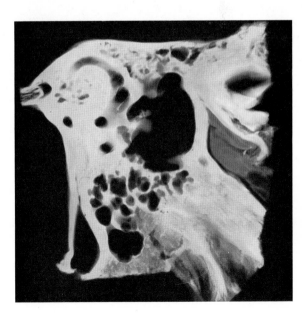

6.25 Microradiograph of macrosection seen in Fig. 6.21 and 6.23.

Sagittal Sections

Figures 6.26–6.31 reveal the structures in a 2 mm thick sagittal section of a right adult temporal bone immediately medial to Fig. 6.20–6.25.

The section crosses the anterior portion of the middle ear and exposes the epi-, meso-, and hypotympanic portions of the middle ear.

The tensor tympani canal protrudes into the middle ear just below the facial nerve.

The anterior portion of the stapes footplate and the anterior crus lie in the anterior part of the oval window niche.

The promontory with the scala vestibuli and tympani lies anterior to the vestibule. The section exposes the round window niche and membrane.

The utricle stretches across the vestibule. Anterosuperiorly the utricular macula connects with the superior vestibular nerve.

The utricle joins the crus commune posterior and the ampullated end of the posterior semicircular canal inferior.

The bony vestibule narrows posteriorly toward the crus commune, which in turn branches to form the non-ampullated limbs of the posterior and superior semicircular canals.

On the posterior aspect, the endolymphatic sac enters the vestibular aqueduct. The aqueduct extends to the vestibule medial to the crus commune.

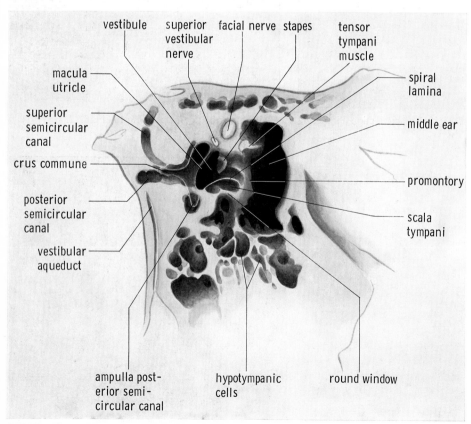

6.26 Drawing of structures seen in Fig. 6.27 to 6.31.

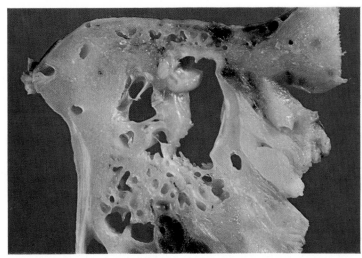

6.27   Photograph of lateral surface of the sagittal macrosection immediately medial to Fig. 6.23.

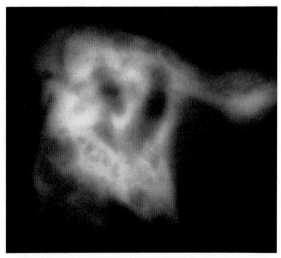

6.28   Tomograph corresponding to Fig. 6.27.

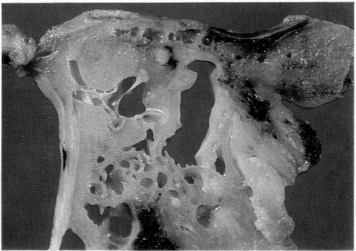

6.29   Photograph of medial surface of sagittal macrosection Fig. 6.27. Reversed photographically.

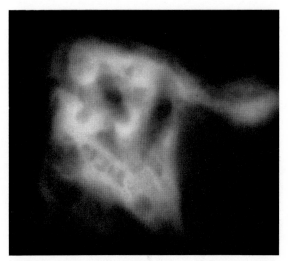

6.30   Tomograph corresponding to Fig. 6.29.

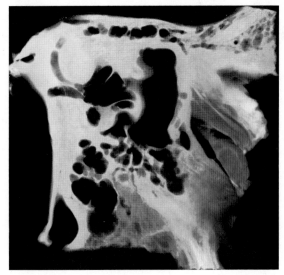

6.31   Microradiograph of macrosection seen in Fig. 6.27 and 6.29.

Sagittal Sections

Figures 6.32–6.37 reveal the structures in a 2 mm thick sagittal section of a right adult temporal bone immediately medial to Fig. 6.26–6.31.

The middle ear narrows near the eustachian tube opening. The tensor tympani canal lies in the superior portion of the middle ear.

Within the thickness of the section the facial nerve courses from the fundus of the internal auditory canal to the geniculate ganglion.

The scala tympani and the smaller scala vestibuli of the first portion of the basal turn of the cochlea lie anterior to the saccule which occupies the spherical recess of the vestibule. The medial surface of the section exposes portions of the middle and apical coils of the cochlea (Fig. 6.35).

The saccule, medial portions of the utricle and membranous crus commune lie on the medial wall of the bony vestibule. A portion of the bony superior semicircular canal passes upwards from the crus commune.

The vestibular aqueduct curves around the medial portion of the crus commune within the thickness of the section.

The fundus of the internal auditory canal lies posterior to the cochlea on the medial surface of the section (Fig. 6.35 and 6.36). The fundus contains portions of the superior and inferior vestibular and facial nerves.

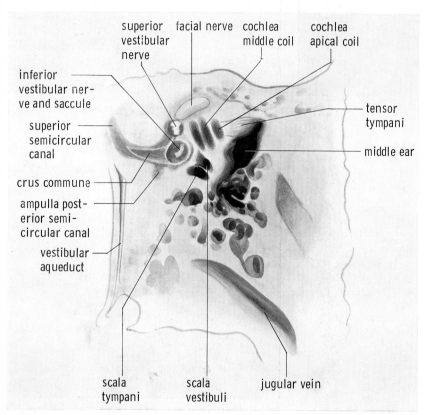

6.32 Drawing of structures seen in Fig. 6.33 to 6.37.

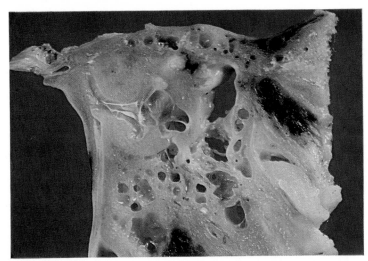

6.33 Photograph of lateral surface of the sagittal macrosection imme-diately medial to Fig. 6.29.

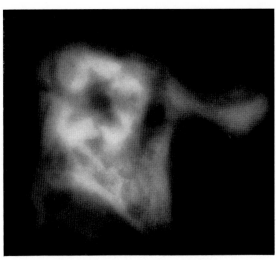

6.34 Tomograph corresponding to Fig. 6.33.

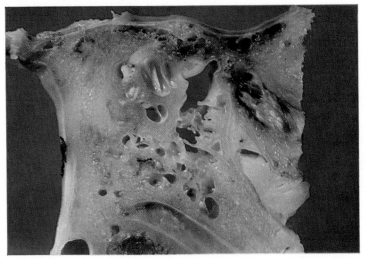

6.35 Photograph of medial surface of sagittal macrosection Fig. 6.33. Reversed photographically.

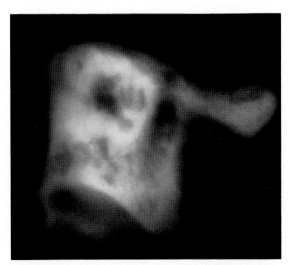

6.36 Tomograph corresponding to Fig. 6.35.

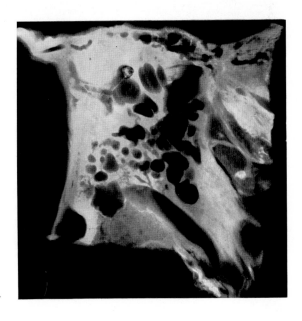

6.37 Microradiograph of macrosection seen in Fig. 6.33 and 6.35.

Sagittal Sections

Figures 6.38–6.43 show the structures in a 2 mm thick sagittal section of a right adult temporal bone immediately medial to Fig. 6.32–6.37.

The tensor tympani canal protrudes into the eustachian portion of the middle ear.

The section exposes the modiolus and three turns of the cochlea. The modiolus is radiolucent and does not appear in the tomographs.

The lateral portion of the internal auditory meatus contains sections of the facial and acoustic nerves.

The carotid artery lies anterior and inferior to the cochlea, while the jugular fossa passes along the inferior surface of the section.

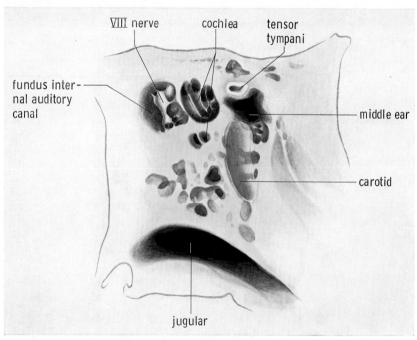

6.38 Drawing of structures seen in Fig. 6.39 to 6.43.

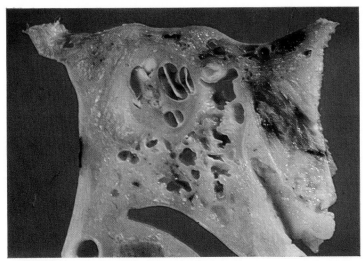

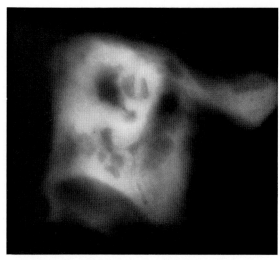

6.39   Photograph of lateral surface of the sagittal macrosection immediately medial to Fig. 6.35.

6.40   Tomograph corresponding to Fig. 6.39.

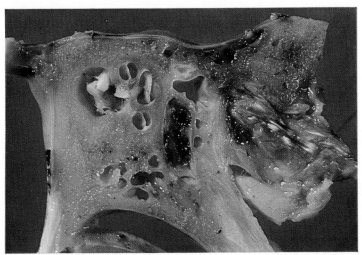

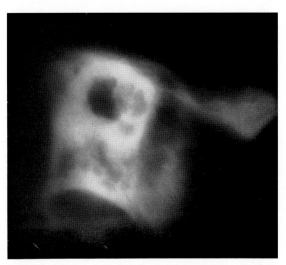

6.41   Photograph of medial surface of sagittal macrosection Fig. 6.39.
Reversed photographically.

6.42   Tomograph correspondingt to Fig. 6.41.

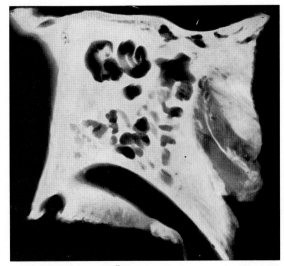

6.43   Microradiograph of macrosection seen in Fig. 6.39
and 6.41.

Sagittal Sections

Figures 6.44–6.49 show the structures contained in a 2 mm thick sagittal section of a right adult temporal bone immediately medial to Fig. 6.38–6.43.
The tensor tympani is in the middle ear portion of the eustachian tube.

The carotid artery courses between the eustachian tube and the cochlea. Parts of the basal and middle coils of the cochlea lie anterior to the internal auditory meatus, while the jugular fossa forms the inferior margin of the section.

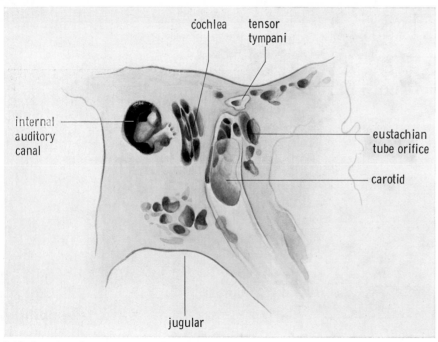

6.44 Drawing of structures seen in Fig. 6.45 to 6.49.

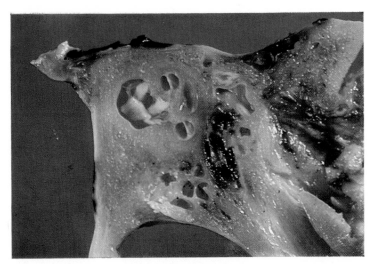

6.45 Photograph of lateral surface of the sagittal macrosection immediately medial to Fig. 6.41.

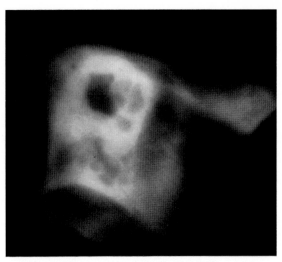

6.46 Tomograph corresponding to Fig. 6.45.

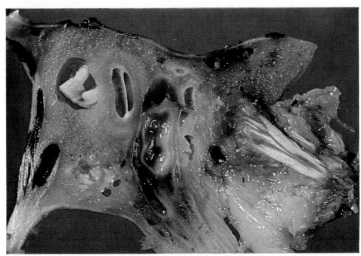

6.47 Photograph of medial surface of sagittal macrosection Fig. 6.45. Reversed photographically.

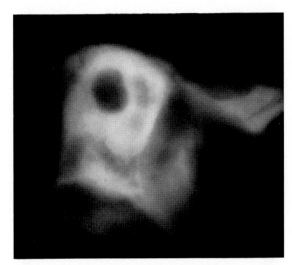

6.48 Tomograph corresponding to Fig. 6.47.

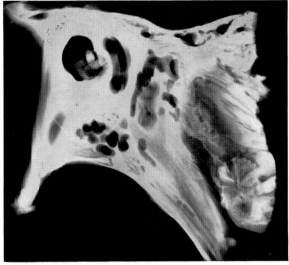

6.49 Microradiograph of macrosection seen in Fig. 6.45 and 6.47.

Sagittal Sections

Figures 6.50–6.55 show the structures in a 2 mm thick sagittal section of a right adult temporal bone immediately medial to Fig. 6.44–6.49.

The section exposes the bony isthmus of the eustachian tube, and a small portion of tubal cartilage. The tensor tympani muscle lies above.

A small portion of the basal turn of the cochlea remains in the section. The carotid artery is anterior to the cochlea and the porus of the internal auditory canal posterior. The jugular fossa forms the inferior contour of the section.

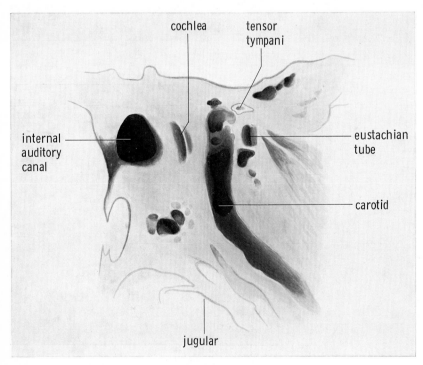

6.50 Drawing of structures seen in Fig. 6.51 to 6.55.

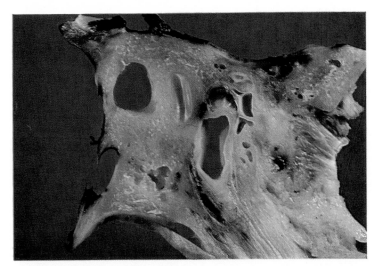

6.51 Photograph of lateral surface of the sagittal macrosection immediately medial to Fig. 6.47.

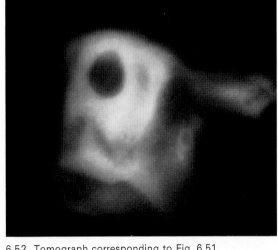

6.52 Tomograph corresponding to Fig. 6.51.

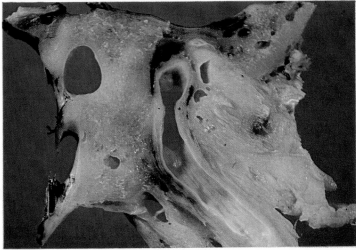

6.53 Photograph of medial surface of sagittal macrosection Fig. 6.51. Reversed photographically.

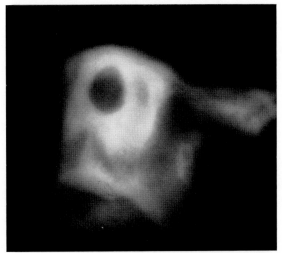

6.54 Tomograph corresponding to Fig. 6.53.

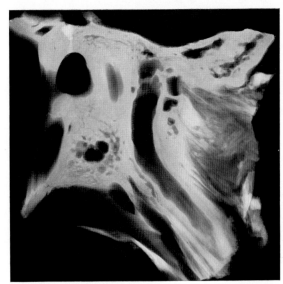

6.55 Microradiograph of macrosection seen in Fig. 6.51 and 6.53.

Chapter 7 Longitudinal Projection of the Petrous Pyramid (Stenvers) and Sections

The longitudinal projection is useful for the evaluation of the petrous pyramid and inner ear structures, particularly the round window, cochlea, posterior semicircular canal and carotid canal. The internal auditory canal is foreshortened as a result of the angulation of the long axis of the canal to the plane of section, but the porus of the canal is visualized on face. This view is unsatisfactory for the study of the external auditory canal and middle ear cavity.

We seldom use the longitudinal projection except for lesions extending to the petrous apex and for fractures of the petrous pyramids. To visualize the plane of fracture at right angles to the plane of section, different projections 45° apart should be obtained.

The longitudinal projection is obtained with the patient supine on the table. The head is rotated 45° toward the opposite side of the ear being examined (Fig. 7.1).

In this atlas, the isolated temporal bones were positioned with the vertical plane through the long axis of the petrous pyramid parallel to the plane of the film.

Nine consecutive sections of the left temporal bone are shown, each 2 mm thick. The photographs of the posterior aspect of each section have been reversed to facilitate comparison with the corresponding tomograms and microradiographs which are included.

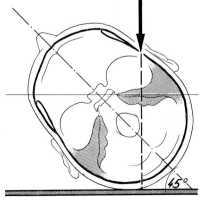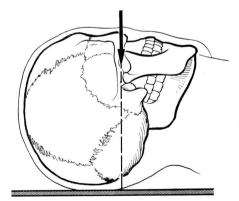

7.1 Longitudinal Projection (Stenvers), head position. The sagittal plane of the skull is rotated 45° towards the opposite side to be examined. The long axis of the petrous pyramid is parallel to the film plane. The arrows indicate the position of the centering point on the surface of the head.

Longitudinal Sections (Stenvers)

These first illustrations (Fig. 7.2–7.7) show the structures in a 2 mm thick, longitudinal section of a left adult temporal bone. The section exposes the external auditory canal and epitympanum in the lateral portion of the bone, and the eustachean tube medially.

Mastoid air cells surround the epitympanum. The section transects the superior portion of the tympanic membrane at the short process of the malleus. Portions of the malleus head and incus body lie in the epitympanum.

The eustachian tube portion of the middle ear extends anteriorly and narrows markedly at the isthmus where the cartilagenous portion of the eustachian tube attaches. The tensor tympani muscle and canal stretch along the upper portion of the eustachian tube.

The tomographs visualize the bony segment of the eustachean tube rather poorly, and the cartilage of the tube is radiolucent.

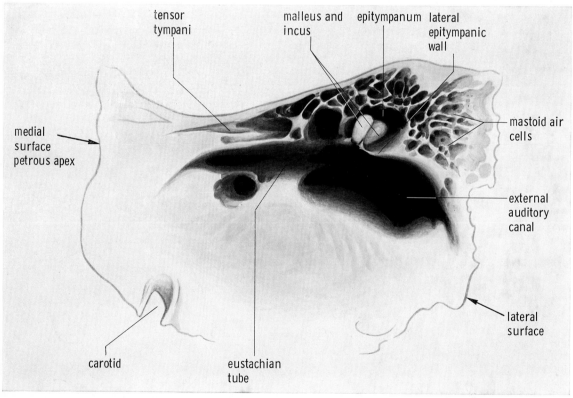

7.2   Drawing of structures seen in Fig. 7.3 to 7.7.

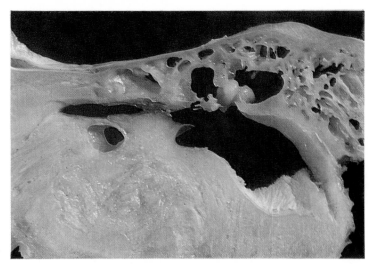

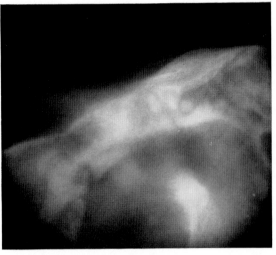

7.3 Photograph of anterior surface of a Stenvers macrosection at the level of the external auditory canal and epitympanum.

7.4   Tomograph corresponding to Fig. 7.3.

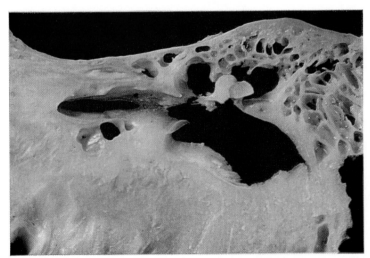

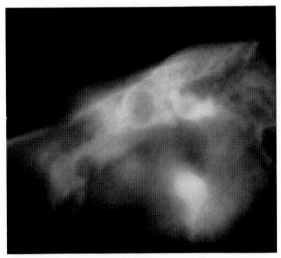

7.5 Photograph of posterior surface of Stenvers macrosection Fig. 7.3. Reversed photographically.

7.6 Tomograph corresponding to Fig. 7.5.

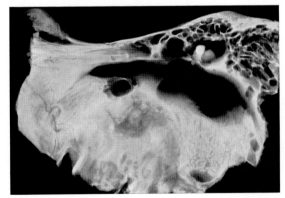

7.7 Microradiograph of macrosection seen in Fig. 7.3 and 7.5.

Longitudinal Sections (Stenvers)

Figures 7.8–7.13 demonstrate the structures contained in a 2 mm thick longitudinal section of a left adult temporal bone immediately posterior to Fig. 7.2–7.7. Mastoid air cells surround the epitympanum, which contains the incus body and a thin slice of the malleus head. The incus short process rests in the fossa incudis. A thin strip of the tympanic membrane demarcates the external and middle ears.

The eustachian portion of the middle ear seems to end bluntly below the tensor tympani canal. In the tomographs two thin parallel lines passing medially represent the tensor tympani canal.

The carotid artery appears in the apical portion of the section. The jugular fossa appears just lateral to the carotid.

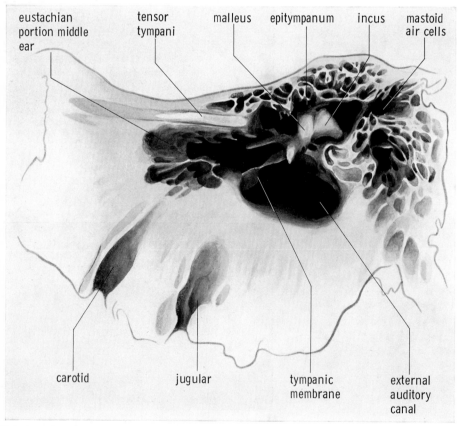

7.8 Drawing of structures seen in Fig. 7.9 to 7.13.

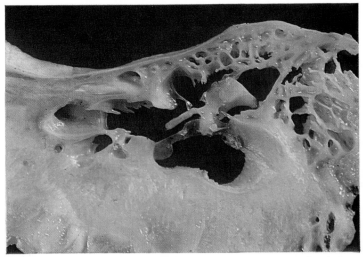

7.9 Photograph of anterior surface of the Stenvers macrosection immediately posterior to Fig. 7.5.

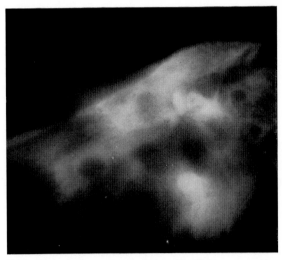

7.10 Tomograph corresponding to Fig. 7.9

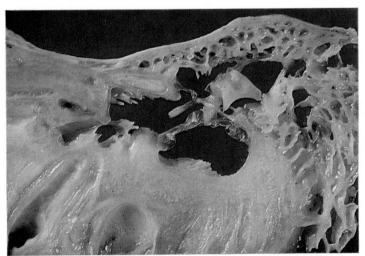

7.11 Photograph of posterior surface of Stenvers macrosection Fig. 7.9. Reversed photographically.

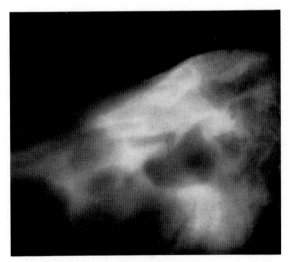

7.12 Tomograph corresponding to Fig. 7.11.

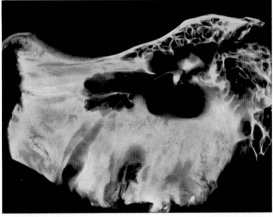

7.13 Microradiograph of macrosection seen in Fig. 7.9 and 7.11.

Longitudinal Sections (Stenvers)

Figures 7.14–7.19 demonstrate the structures contained in a 2 mm thick longitudinal section of a left adult temporal bone immediately posterior to Fig. 7.8–7.13.

Mastoid air cells surround the mastoid antrum and epitympanum.

The tensor tympani muscle becomes tendinous at the cochleariform process and crosses the middle ear to attach to the neck of the malleus.

The malleus handle is attached to a section of the tympanic membrane which fans out inferior.

In the tomographs, the long process of the incus parallels the malleus handle. The long process is absent in the sections and microradiograph.

A small portion of the geniculate ganglion is present on the posterior surface of the section just above the tensor tympani muscle and cochleariform process (Fig. 7.17).

The entire arch of the carotid artery occupies the medial portion of the section. The jugular fossa appears inferior and lateral to the carotid.

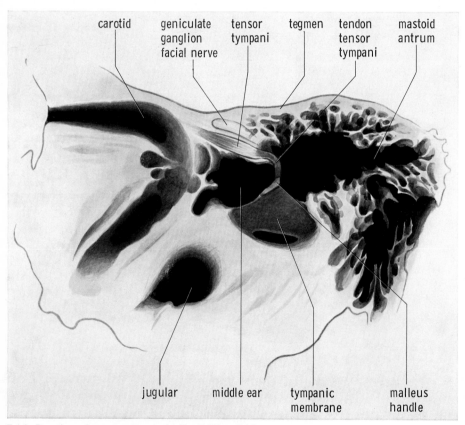

7.14 Drawing of structures seen in Fig. 7.15 to 7.19.

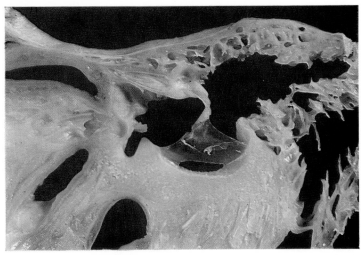

7.15 Photograph of anterior surface of the Stenvers macrosection immediately posterior to Fig. 7.11.

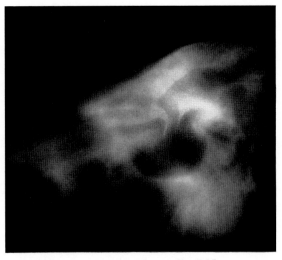

7.16 Tomograph corresponding to Fig. 7.15.

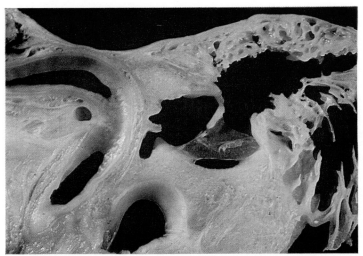

7.17 Photograph of posterior surface of Stenvers macrosection Fig. 7.15.
Reversed photographically.

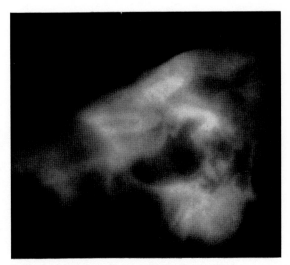

7.18 Tomograph corresponding to Fig. 7.17.

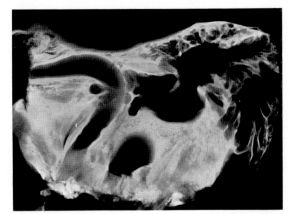

7.19 Microradiograph of macrosection seen in Fig. 7.15
and 7.17.

Longitudinal Sections (Stenvers)

Figures 7.20–7.25 reveal the structures contained in a 2 mm thick longitudinal section of a left adult temporal bone immediately posterior to Fig. 7.14–7.19.

Mastoid air cells extend from the antrum. The facial nerve stretches from the geniculate ganglion laterally below the prominence of the horizontal semicircular canal.

A thin slice of the promontory of the cochlea forms the medial wall of the middle ear.

The apex of the cochlea lies just lateral to the arch of the carotid artery. The helicotrema appears as a small foramen in the center of the cochlea (Fig. 7.23).

The jugular fossa bounds the inferior portion of the middle ear.

The superior semicircular canal begins to appear in the tomographs.

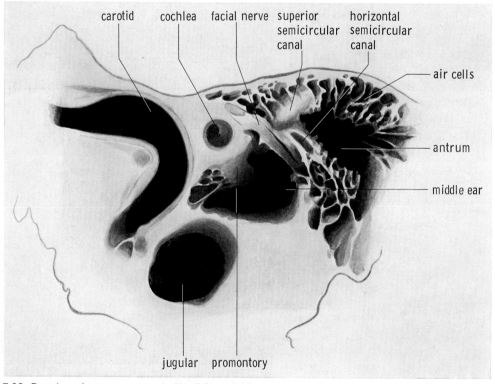

7.20 Drawing of structures seen in Fig. 7.21 to 7.25.

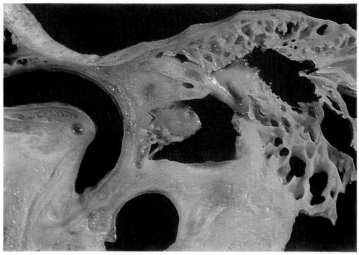

7.21 Photograph of anterior surface of the Stenvers macrosection immediately posterior to Fig. 7.17.

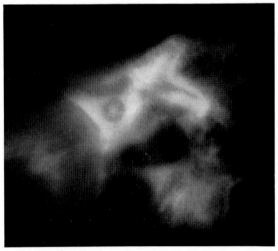

7.22 Tomograph corresponding to Fig. 7.21.

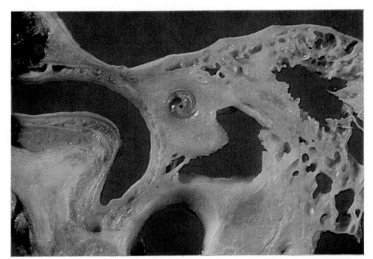

7.23 Photograph of posterior surface of Stenvers macrosection Fig. 7.21. Reversed photographically.

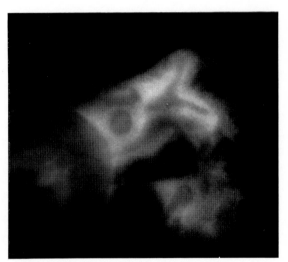

7.24 Tomograph corresponding to Fig. 7.23.

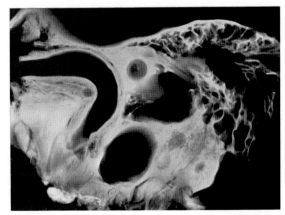

7.25 Microradiograph of macrosection seen in Fig. 7.21 and 7.23.

Longitudinal Sections (Stenvers)

Figures 7.26–7.31 expose the structures in a 2 mm thick longitudinal section of a left adult temporal bone immediately posterior to Fig. 7.20–7.25.

The section exposes the mastoid air cells and the posterior portion of the middle ear. The horizontal and superior semicircular canals open into the vestibule.

The membranous ampullas of the horizontal and superior canals with their cristae are in their respective bony canals. The macula of the utricle occupies the lumen of the vestibule just superior to the anterior portion of the stapes footplate (Fig. 7.29).

There are three segments of the facial nerve in this section. The proximal portion of the nerve is above the cochlea. The horizontal portion lies under the horizontal semicircular canal, and the vertical portion descends from the pyramidal turn.

The stapes superstructure fills the oval window niche. The tendon of the stapedius muscle passes to the stapes neck from the pyramidal eminence.

Three coils of the cochlea are present. The lamina spiralis separates the scala vestibuli from the scala tympani. The plane of the posterior surface of the section is parallel to and almost coincides with the plane of the spiral lamina. Because of this relationship, the scala tympani surface of the spiral lamina appears on face for almost the entire length of the basal coil (Fig. 7.29).

The slight indentation of the lower margin of the promontory represents the lateral or external lip of the round window niche (Fig. 7.29, 7.30, 7.31).

The carotid artery again appears medially, and the jugular fossa inferior.

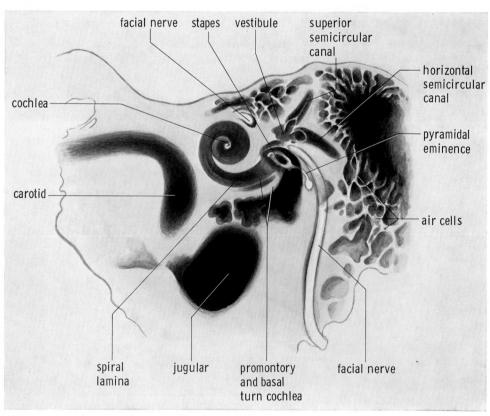

7.26 Drawing of structures seen in Fig. 7.27 to 7.31.

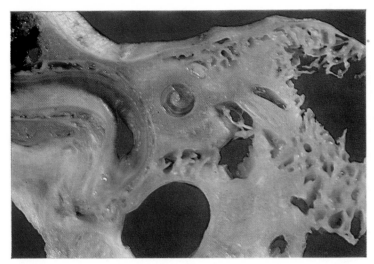

7.27 Photograph of anterior surface of the Stenvers macrosection immediately posterior to Fig. 7.23.

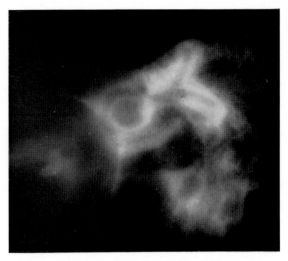

7.28 Tomograph corresponding to Fig. 7.27.

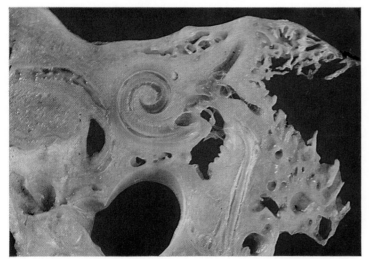

7.29 Photograph of posterior surface of Stenvers macrosection Fig. 7.27.
Reversed photographically.

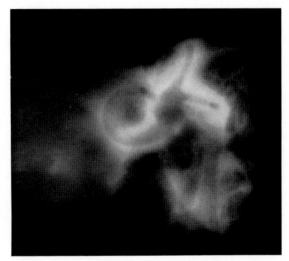

7.30 Tomograph corresponding to Fig. 7.29.

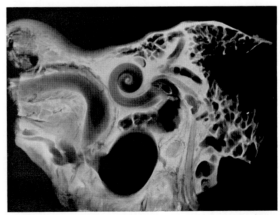

7.31 Microradiograph of macrosection seen in Fig. 7.27
and 7.29.

Longitudinal Sections (Stenvers)

Figures 7.32–7.37 expose the structures in a 2 mm thick longitudinal section of a left adult temporal bone immediately posterior to Fig. 7.26–7.31.

Mastoid air cells lie lateral to the superior and horizontal semicircular canals and to the descending portion of the facial nerve.

The membranous ampullas of the superior and horizontal canals open into the utricle. The macula of the utricle crosses the upper portion of the vestibule in close relation to the posterior portion of the stapes footplate. The saccule lies on the medial wall of the vestibule (Fig. 7.33 and 7.35).

A segment of the promontory separates the oval window above and the round window below (Fig. 7.30 and 7.34). The lumen of the scala tympani appears on the anterior surface of the section (Fig. 7.33). Just above the round window a cross section of the spiral lamina, basilar membrane, and spiral ligament separates the scala tympani from the scala vestibuli. The round window membrane closes the scala tympani in the round window niche.

The cochlear aqueduct opens into a small pore on the posterior wall of the scala tympani near the round window membrane.

The small segment of the middle ear, located between the labyrinth windows and the descending portion of the facial nerve represents the sinus tympani.

The proximal portion of the facial nerve lies above the cochlea. Just lateral to this portion of the facial nerve, the superior vestibular nerve passes to the macula of the utricle.

The fundus of the internal auditory canal and the base of the modiolus are on the posterior surface of the section (Fig. 7.35).

The jugular fossa is inferior.

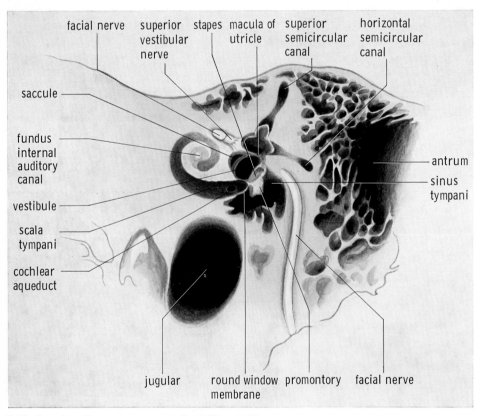

7.32 Drawing of structures seen in Fig. 7.33 to 7.37.

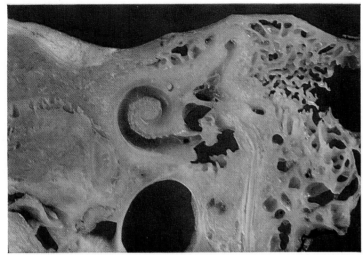

7.33 Photograph of anterior surface of the Stenvers macrosection immediately posterior to Fig. 7.29.

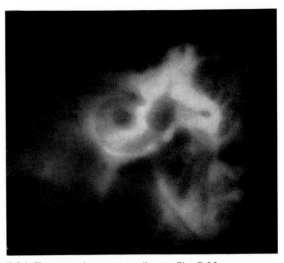

7.34 Tomograph corresponding to Fig. 7.33.

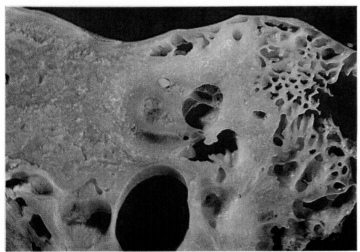

7.35 Photograph of posterior surface of Stenvers macrosection Fig. 7.33 Reversed photographically.

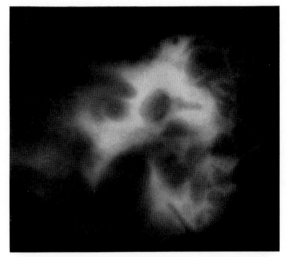

7.36 Tomograph corresponding to Fig. 7.35.

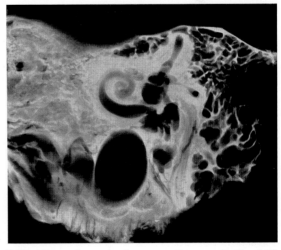

7.37 Microradiograph of macrosection seen in Fig. 7.33 and 7.35.

Figures 7.38–7.43 reveal the structures in a 2 mm thick longitudinal section of a left adult temporal bone immediately posterior to Fig. 7.32–7.37.

Mastoid air cells surround the horizontal and superior semicircular canals. In the tomographs, the posterior semicircular canal begins to appear (Fig. 7.42).

The vestibule is lateral to the fundus of the internal auditory canal. The crista falciformis divides the internal auditory canal into two unequal compartments. The superior, smaller compartment contains the facial and superior vestibular nerves; the cochlear and the inferior vestibular nerves occupy the inferior compartment.

The saccular macula appears on the vestibular wall on the anterior surface of the section (Fig. 7.39). The inferior vestibular nerve passes to the saccule from the fundus of the internal auditory canal within the thickness of the section (Fig. 7.43).

The jugular fossa lies inferior.

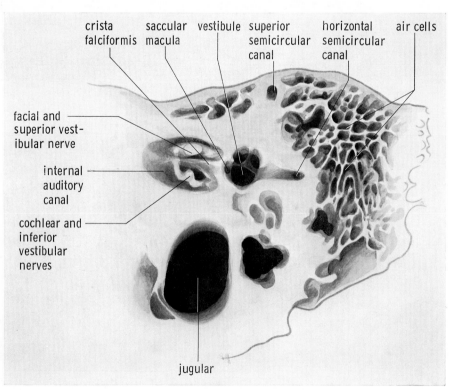

7.38 Drawing of structures seen in Fig. 7.39 to 7.43.

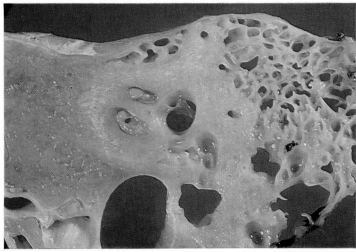

7.39 Photograph of anterior surface of the Stenvers macrosection immediately posterior to Fig. 7.35.

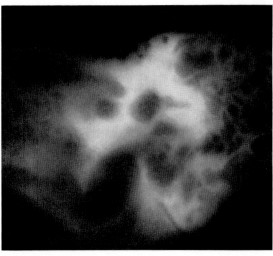

7.40 Tomograph corresponding to Fig. 7.39.

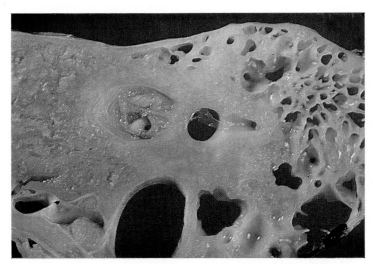

7.41 Photograph of posterior surface of Stenvers macrosection Fig. 7.39. Reversed photographically.

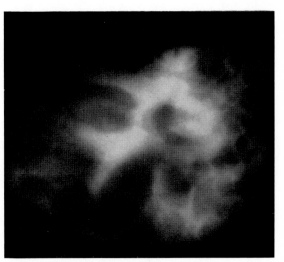

7.42 Tomograph corresponding to Fig. 7.41.

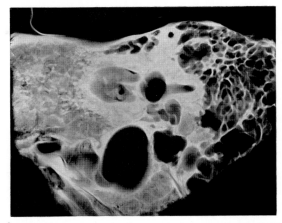

7.43 Microradiograph of macrosection seen in Fig. 7.39 and 7.41.

Longitudinal Sections (Stenvers)

Figures 7.44–7.49 demonstrate the structures in a 2 mm thick longitudinal section of a left adult temporal bone immediately posterior to Fig. 7.38–7.43.

Mastoid air cells are lateral to the horizontal, superior, and posterior semicircular canals.

The ampulla of the posterior semicircular canal enters the inferior portion of the vestibule. Portions of the membranous labyrinth occupy the lumina of the vestibule and semicircular canals.

The nerve to the posterior semicircular canal leaves the inferior compartment of the internal auditory canal at the foramen singulare and stretches towards the posterior semicircular canal.

The jugular fossa is inferior.

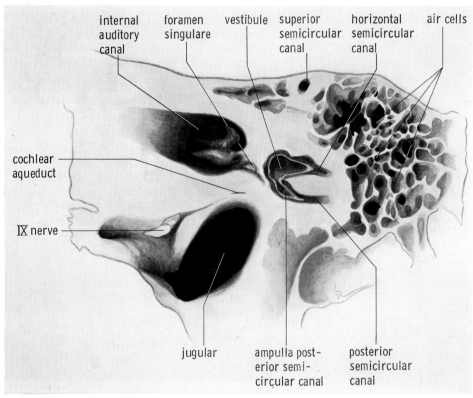

7.44 Drawing of structures seen in Fig. 7.45 to 7.49.

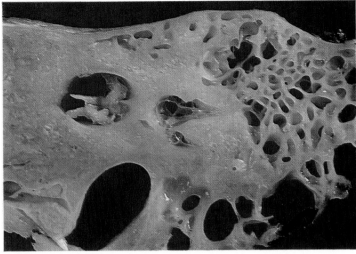

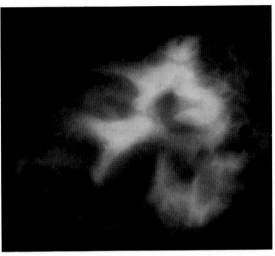

7.45 Photograph of anterior surface of the Stenvers macrosection immediately posterior to Fig. 7.41.

7.46 Tomograph corresponding to Fig. 7.45.

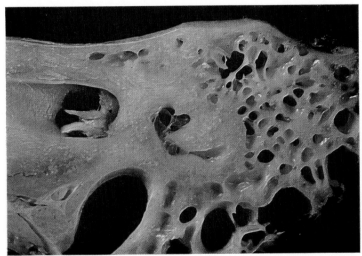

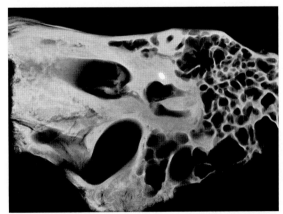

7.47 Photograph of posterior surface of Stenvers macrosection Fig. 7.45. Reversed photographically.

7.48 Tomograph corresponding to Fig. 7.47.

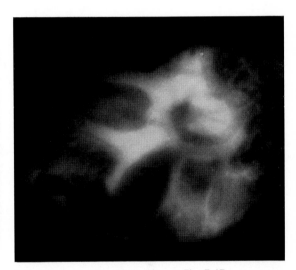

7.49 Microradiograph of macrosection seen in Fig. 7.45 and 7.47.

Longitudinal Sections (Stenvers)

Figures 7.50–7.55 represent the structures in a 2 mm thick longitudinal section of a left adult temporal bone immediately posterior to Fig. 7.44–7.49.
Mastoid air cells occupy the lateral portion of the section.
Within the thickness of the section, the posterior semicircular canal arches to the crus commune where it joins the posterior limb of the superior semicircular canal.

The porus of the internal auditory canal has a sharp lateral margin formed by the lip of the posterior wall.
The jugular fossa lies inferior and the cochlear aqueduct opens into the neural portion of the jugular foramen.

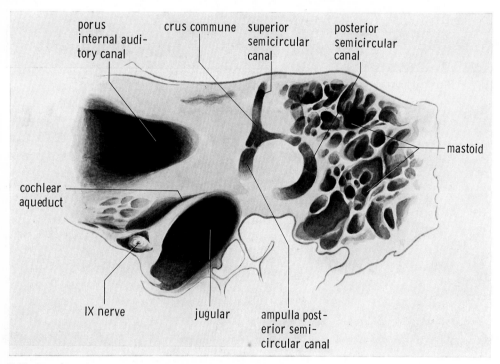

7.50 Drawing of structures seen in Fig. 7.51 to 7.55.

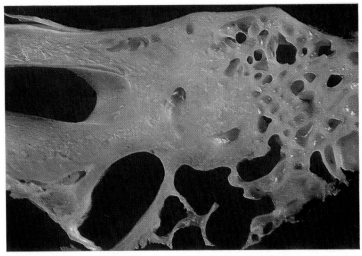

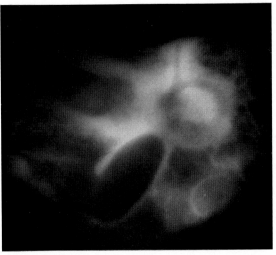

7.51 Photograph of anterior surface of the Stenvers macrosection immediately posterior to Fig. 7.47.

7.52 Tomograph corresponding to Fig. 7.51.

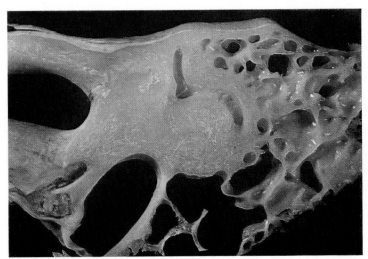

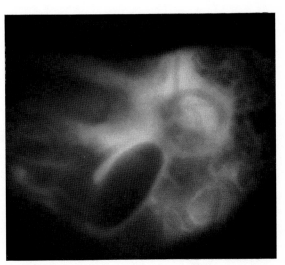

7.53 Photograph of posterior surface of Stenvers macrosection Fig. 7.51. Reversed photographically.

7.54 Tomograph corresponding to Fig. 7.53.

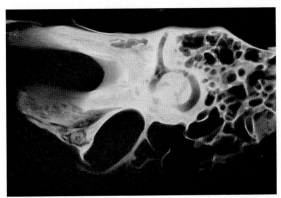

7.55 Microradiograph of macrosection seen in Fig. 7.51 and 7.53.

Pathological Findings in the Temporal Bone

Chapter 8   Congenital Anomalies

A radiographic study is essential in the evaluation of the ear with congenital anomalies. Otoscopy is difficult or impossible in cases of partial or complete atresia of the external auditory canal. Audiometric assessment in the very young is often unreliable.

Conventional radiography is of limited value in congenital anomalies except for the evaluation of the degree of development of the mastoid. A tomographic examination should be performed for proper evaluation. The tomographic study should be carried out in at least two projections, coronal and sagittal, with sections 1 or 2 mm apart. Horizontal and semiaxial sections, the latter for the evaluation of the oval window, are taken when indicated.

A proper tomographic study can provide the surgeon with the following information of basic importance in the decision of whether to perform corrective surgery and of what type of surgery to perform:

1) Degree and type of abnormality of the tympanic bone. The anomalies may range from a minor deformity of the external auditory canal to complete agenesis;

2) Degree and localization of development of the mastoid cells and mastoid antrum;

3) Position of the sigmoid sinus and jugular bulb. It is not uncommon to demonstrate a deep jugular fossa protruding from below into the hypotympanic or tympanic cavity. The jugular bulb may be covered by a thin bony shell or bulge into the middle ear cavity without a bony cover;

4) Degree of development and aeration of the middle ear cavity;

5) Condition of the ossicular chain. The tomographs will reveal information about the size, shape, fusion, and fixation of the ossicles;

6) Status of the labyrinthine windows;

7) Development and route of the facial nerve canal. The vertical portion of the facial nerve canal may be grossly ectopic and run horizontally outward;

8) Relationship of the meninges to the mastoid and petrous ridge. A low lying dura is frequently encountered as the middle cranial fossa deepens to form a large groove lateral to the labyrinth;

9) Development and morphology of the inner ear structures. Congenital abnormalities involving only the membranous portion of the labyrinth are not demonstrable radiographically. Anomalies involving both the membranous and bony labyrinth will appear tomographically.

Congenital malformations may involve the sound conducting system or the cochlear-vestibular, perceptive apparatus. Anomalies of the conducting apparatus are more frequent than inner ear malformations.

Most commonly the external auditory canal is involved in varying degrees from mild narrowing to complete atresia. The ossicles may be fused together and the malleus neck fixed to the atretic plate of the external canal.

Congenital anolmalies of the inner ear structures range from complete agenesis or aplasia of the Michel type to hypoplasia or dysplasia of one or more structures. The single most common radiographically demonstrable anomaly of the inner ear involves the horizontal semicircular canal. In this defect the horizontal canal forms a single large pouch extending laterally from the vestibule. An isolated malformation of this type does not necessarily involve the membranous labyrinth, since in approximately 50% of these cases the hearing and the caloric tests are normal.

Congenital Anomalies of the Temporal Bone

An example of a temporal bone with multiple anomalies of the sound conduction and perceptive systems is shown in Fig. 8.1–8.46. These sections show the right temporal bone of a six month infant who died from multiple congenital defects of the heart and great vessels. There was microtia on the right side associated with right facial paralysis.

Coronal sections, 2 mm thick, reveal agenesis of the external auditory canal, severe hypoplasia of the middle ear and ossicles, anomalies of the inner ear, and a rudimentary facial nerve.

Figures 8.1–8.6 cross the most anterior part of the malformed middle ear cleft and the anterior, horizontal portion of the carotid artery.

A rudimentary ossicular mass lies in the middle ear cleft. Mesenchymal tissue surrounds the ossicular mass and fills the middle ear cleft. The middle ear cleft is displaced laterally and anteriorly.

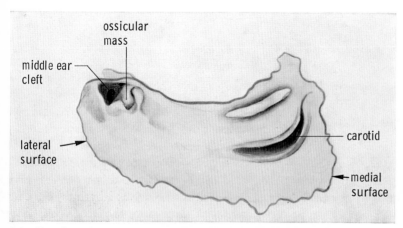

8.1   Drawing of structures and pathology seen in Fig. 8.2 to 8.6.

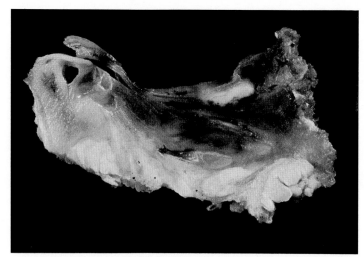

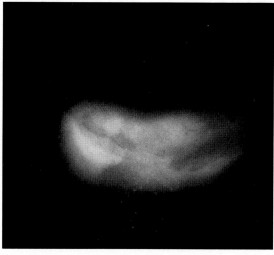

8.2   Photograph of anterior surface of a coronal macrosection at the level of the malformed middle ear cleft and the carotid artery.

8.3   Tomograph corresponding to Fig. 8.2.

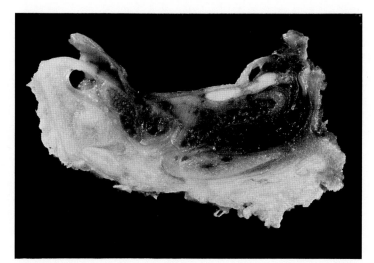

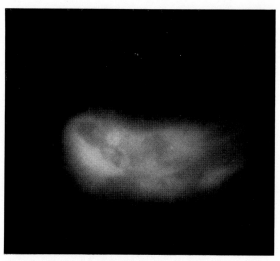

8.4   Photograph of posterior surface of coronal macrosection Fig. 8.2. Reversed photographically.

8.5   Tomograph corresponding to Fig. 8.9.

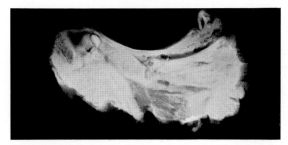

8.6   Microradiograph of coronal macrosection seen in Fig. 8.2 and 8.9.

Congenital Anomalies of the Temporal Bone

Figures 8.7–8.12 show the congenital anomalies in a 2 mm thick, coronal section of the same right temporal bone, 2 mm posterior to Fig. 8.1–8.6. The intervening 2 mm thick tissue section is omitted.

The section crosses the anterior margin of the cochlea and the vertical segment of the carotid canal.

The middle ear cleft is extremely narrow and filled with mesenchymal tissue. The external auditory canal is absent.

An extremely small facial nerve canal lies above the cochlea. There is no neural tissue within the punctate lumen of the canal. The facial nerve appears to terminate at this area, normally the site of the geniculate ganglion.

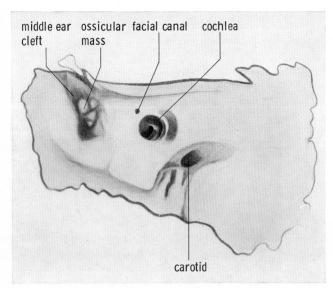

8.7   Drawing of structures and pathology seen in Fig. 8.8 to 8.12.

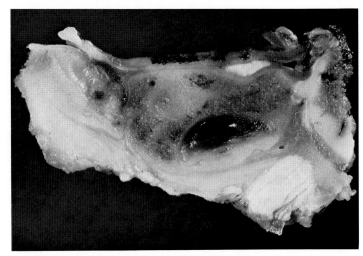

8.8   Photograph of anterior surface of the coronal macrosection 2 mm posterior to Fig. 8.4.

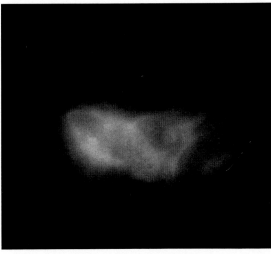

8.9   Tomograph corresponding to Fig. 8.8.

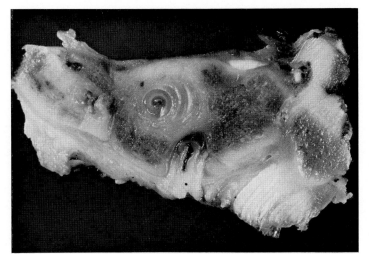

8.10   Photograph of posterior surface of coronal macrosection Fig. 8.8. Reversed photographically.

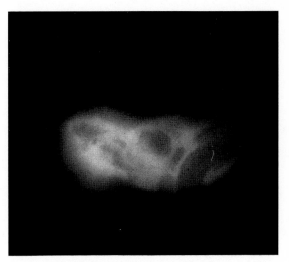

8.11   Tomograph corresponding to Fig. 8.10.

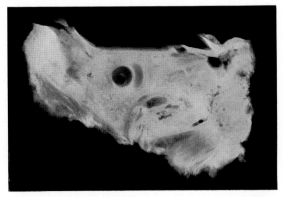

8.12   Microradiograph of coronal macrosection seen in Fig. 8.8 and 8.10.

Congenital Anomalies of the Temporal Bone

Figures 8.13–8.18 show the congenital anomalies in a 2 mm thick, coronal section of the same right temporal bone, immediately posterior to Fig. 8.7–8.12.

The section crosses the cochlea and proximal portion of the carotid canal.

There is no external auditory canal, and the narrow middle ear cleft is filled with mesenchymal tissue.

The small facial nerve canal is adjacent to the upper margin of the cochlea. There is a small amount of neural tissue within the canal lumen. Subsequent sections will show that only the petrous portion of the facial nerve is present in this bone. The geniculate ganglion and more distal portions of the facial nerve are absent. The tensor tympani muscle is missing. The cochlea appears normal.

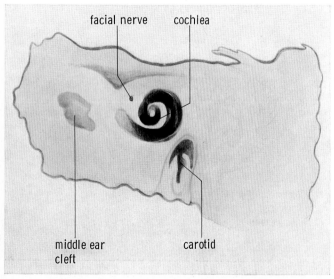

8.13   Drawing of structures and pathology seen in Fig. 9.14 to 8.18.

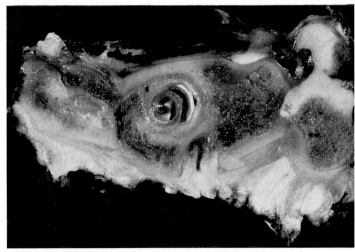

8.14   Photograph of anterior surface of the coronal macrosection immediately posterior to Fig. 8.10.

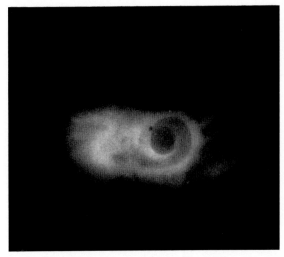

8.15   Tomograph corresponding to Fig. 8.14.

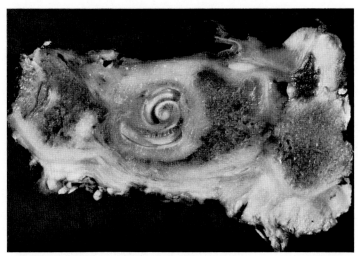

8.16   Photograph of posterior surface of coronal macrosection Fig. 8.14. Reversed photographically.

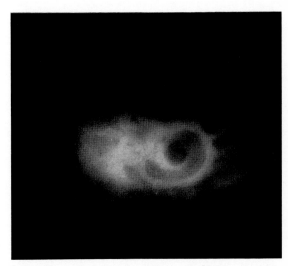

8.17   Tomograph corresponding to Fig. 8.16

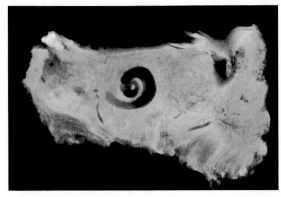

8.18   Microradiograph of coronal macrosection seen in Fig. 8.14 and 8.16.

Congenital Anomalies of the Temporal Bone

Figures 8.19–8.24 show the congenital anomalies in a 2 mm thick, coronal section of the same right temporal bone, immediately posterior to Fig. 8.13–8.18.

The section crosses the cochlea, the fundus of the internal auditory canal, the anterior vestibule, and the ampullated ends of the horizontal and superior semicircular canals.

The external auditory canal is missing, and the middle ear is reduced to a slit. A small rudimentary stapes lies in the narrow and malformed oval window area.

The proximal, petrous segment of the facial nerve lies above the cochlea.

The basal turn of the cochlea coils within the thickness of the section to the round window area.

The ampullated ends of the bony superior and horizontal semicircular canals open into the superior portion of the vestibule on the posterior surface of the section (Fig. 8.22).

The bony horizontal semicircular canal is short and wide and opens into the vestibule throughout its entire extent. Subsequent sections demonstrate that the deformed horizontal semicircular canal forms a single, large pouch lateral to the vestibule.

The membranous superior and horizontal semicircular canals join the utricle. The cristae appear normal. The macula of the utricle is thickened.

The round window membrane closes the scala tympani (Fig. 8.22, 8.23, 8.24).

Segments of the facial and acoustic nerves lie in the fundus of the internal auditory canal above and below the crista falciformis (Fig. 8.22).

The facial nerve in the fundus of the internal auditory canal is very thick, but as it passes into the facial canal it narrows to a thread-like structure.

There is no facial nerve below the horizontal semicircular canal.

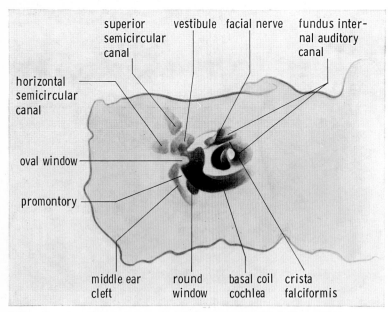

8.19   Drawing of structures and pathology seen in Fig. 8.20 to 8.24.

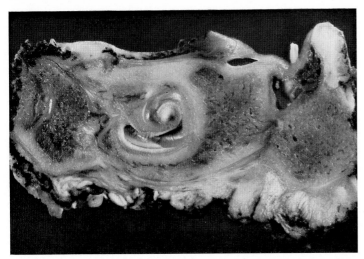

8.20   Photograph of anterior surface of the coronal macrosection immediately posterior to Fig. 8.16.

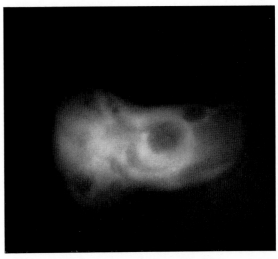

8.21   Tomograph corresponding to Fig. 8.20.

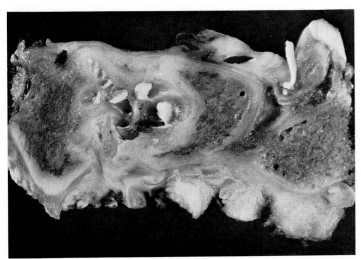

8.22   Photograph of posterior surface of coronal macrosection Fig. 8.20. Reversed photographically.

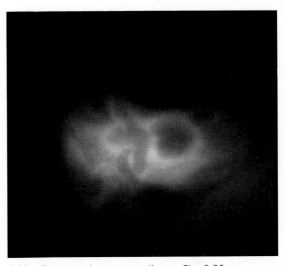

8.23   Tomograph corresponding to Fig. 8.22.

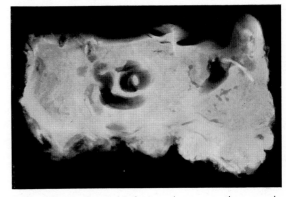

8.24   Microradiograph of coronal macrosection seen in Fig. 8.20 and 8.22.

Congenital Anomalies of the Temporal Bone

Figures 8.25–8.30 show the congenital anomalies in a 2 mm thick, coronal section of the same right temporal bone immediately posterior to Fig. 8.19–8.24

The section crosses the vestibule, the horizontal and superior semicircular canals, and the internal auditory canal.

A small, rudimentary middle ear cleft lies inferior at the level of the round window.

The horizontal canal is widened and shortened and opens into the vestibule throughout its entire length. Actually the horizontal semicircular canal forms a lat-

eral outpouching of the vestibule. The lumen of the superior semicircular canal is wider than normal.

The thickened utricular macula stretches across the vestibule, and the saccule lies on the medial vestibular wall.

The cribriform plate between the internal auditory canal and the vestibule is thickened. The internal auditory canal is unusually wide.

There is no trace of the horizontal portion of the facial nerve. The jugular fossa lies inferior.

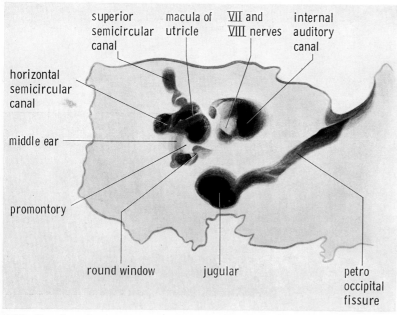

8.25   Drawing of structures and pathology seen in Fig. 8.26 to 8.30.

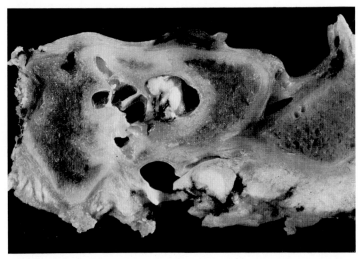

8.26   Photograph of anterior surface of the coronal macrosection immediately posterior to Fig. 8.22.

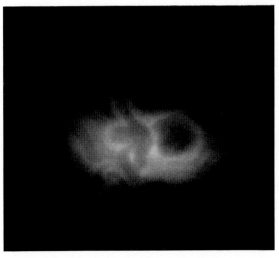

8.27   Tomograph corresponding to Fig. 8.26.

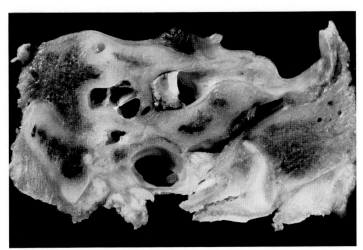

8.28   Photograph of posterior surface of coronal macrosection Fig. 8.26. Reversed photographically.

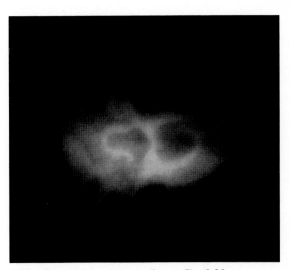

8.29   Tomograph corresponding to Fig. 8.28.

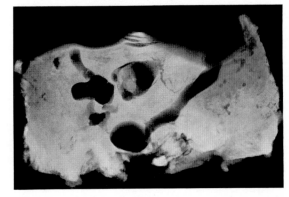

8.30   Microradiograph of coronal macrosection seen in Fig. 8.26 and 8.28.

Congenital Anomalies of the Temporal Bone

Figures 8.31–8.36 show the congenital anomalies in a 2 mm thick, coronal section of the same right temporal bone immediately posterior to Fig. 8.25–8.30.

The section crosses the posterior portion of the deformed horizontal semicircular canal and the posterior wall of the internal auditory canal.

Both the middle ear cleft and mastoid antrum are absent.

The horizontal semicircular canal forms a large lateral outpouching of the posterior portion of the vestibule. On the posterior surface of the section the ampullated end of the posterior semicircular canal enters the vestibule inferior (Fig. 8.34, 8.35). The subarcuate fossa passes through the arch of the superior semicircular canal (Fig. 8.34).

There is no facial nerve; the jugular fossa lies inferior.

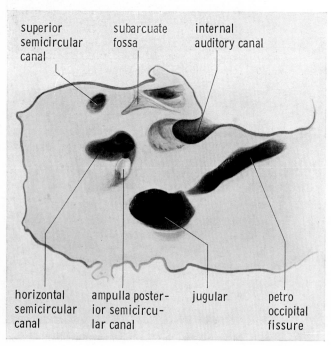

8.31   Drawing of structures and pathology seen in Fig. 8.32 to 8.36.

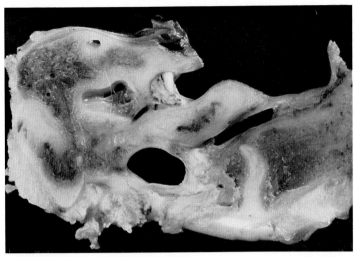

8.32 Photograph of anterior surface of the coronal macrosection immediately posterior to Fig. 8.28.

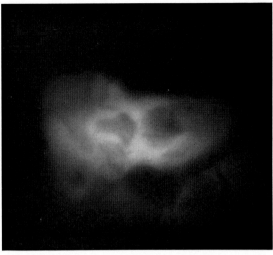

8.33 Tomograph corresponding to Fig. 8.32.

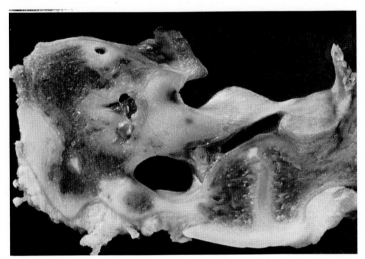

8.34 Photograph of posterior surface of coronal macrosection Fig. 8.32. Reversed photographically.

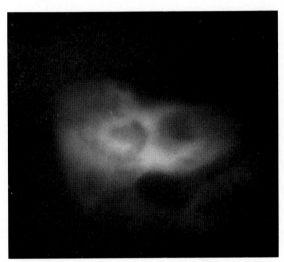

8.35 Tomograph corresponding to Fig. 8.34.

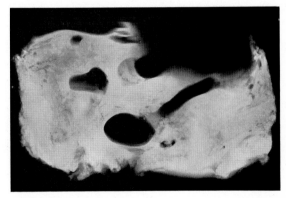

8.36 Microradiograph of coronal macrosection seen in Fig. 8.32 and 8.34.

Congenital Anomalies of the Temporal Bone

Figures 8.37–8.42 show the congenital anomalies in a 2 mm thick, coronal section of the same right temporal bone immediately posterior to Fig. 8.31–8.36.

The section crosses the posterior aspect of the vestibule, the posterior semicircular canal, and the crus commune.

There are no mastoid air cells. The lumen of the loop of the posterior semicircular canal appears wider than normal.

The jugular fossa lies inferior.

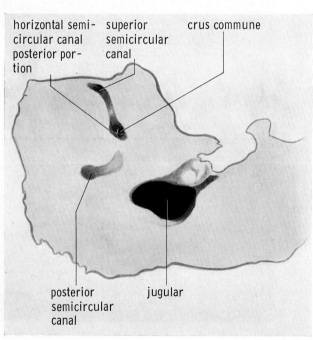

horizontal semi-circular canal posterior portion   superior semicircular canal   crus commune

posterior semicircular canal   jugular

8.37   Drawing of structures and pathology seen in Fig. 8.38 to 8.42.

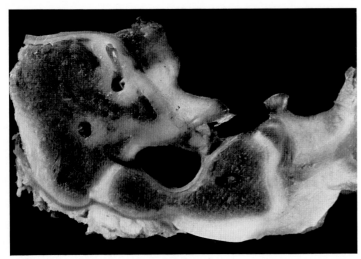

8.38   Photograph of anterior surface of the coronal macrosection immediately posterior to Fig. 8.34.

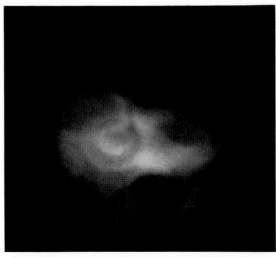

8.39   Tomograph corresponding to Fig. 8.38.

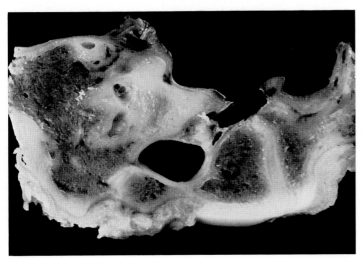

8.40   Photograph of posterior surface of coronal macrosection Fig. 8.38. Reversed photographically.

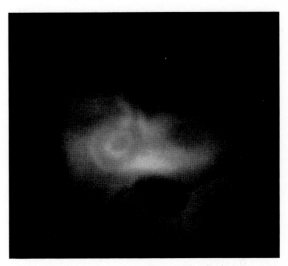

8.41   Tomograph corresponding to Fig. 8.40.

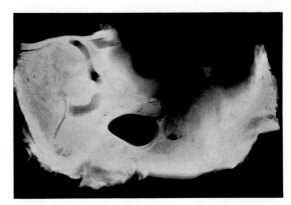

8.42   Microradiograph of coronal macrosection seen in Fig. 8.38 and 8.40.

Congenital Anomalies of the Temporal Bone

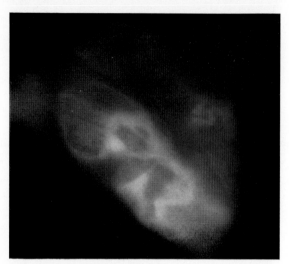

8.43   Horizontal tomograph.

These three consecutive horizontal tomographs are from the same right temporal bone with congenital anomalies as Fig. 8.1–8.42. Figure 8.43 is the most superior section, and the following tomographs 1 mm apart extend inferiorly (Fig. 8.44, 8.45). The external auditory canal is absent. A rudimentary ossicular mass lies in the anterolateral portion of the middle ear cleft. The horizontal semicircular canal has no loop and forms a dilated, lateral outpouching of the vestibule.

The cochlea appears normal, but the internal auditory canal is wider than normal.

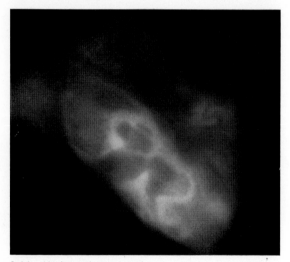

8.44   Horizontal tomograph.

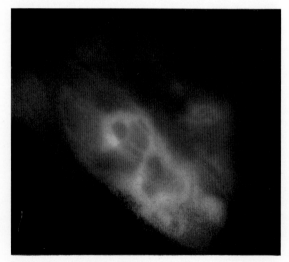

8.45   Horizontal tomograph.

Chapter 9 Inflammatory Processes and Cholesteatoma

Our radiographic study of the middle ear and mastoid for inflammatory processes and cholesteatoma consists of conventional Schüller views of both mastoids and of tomographic sections 2 mm apart in the coronal, sagittal and semiaxial projections. The sagittal tomographic sections extend from the external auditory canal and mastoid to the vestibule of the labyrinth. If the pathologic process is unilateral, only frontal sections of the normal side are obtained for comparison purposes.

Acute and Subacute Inflammatory Proccesses

Acute and subacute inflammatory processes produce a diffuse and homogeneous clouding of the mastoid air cells and middle ear cavity. In the initial stage of the inflammatory process the trabecular pattern of the mastoid is intact, although the trabeculae appear less clear than usual because of the lack of the normal air bone interface due to edema of the mucosa and/or collection of fluid in the air cells. Whenever the infection is not arrested by effective therapy, necrosis of the cell walls develops which may lead to formation of areas of coalescence. Since the radiographic density of serous fluid, blood or pus is identical, the radiologist needs some basic clinical information to reach a correct interpretation of the radiographic findings.

Chronic Inflammation

Chronic inflammatory processes of the middle ear and mastoid cause lytic and sclerotic changes in the trabecular pattern of the mastoid. The finer trabeculae become demineralized and reabsorbed and the primary trabeculae are thickened by apposition of new bone. The proliferative process may progress to a complete bony obliteration of the air cells and to a diffuse sclerosis of the mastoid. This type of inflammatory sclerosis

of a previously pneumatized mastoid must be distinguished from a compact or diploic mastoid in which the pneumatic system never developed.

Osteitic processes may occur in the middle ear cavity and lead to necrosis of the long process of the incus.

In chronic inflammation the mastoid air cells and the middle ear cavity are partially or completely cloudy, but the soft tissue densities are usually less diffuse and homogenous than in acute and subacute processes.

Tympanosclerotic deposits are occasionally demonstrated by tomography. These deposits appear as irregularly calcified plaques or masses which in severe cases may conglobate the entire ossicular chain.

Cholesteatoma

Microscopic otoscopy usually provides the diagnosis of cholesteatoma but gives no concept of the size and extent of the lesion in the mastoid and middle ear. Cholesteatomas characteristically result in erosion or destruction of the structures of the middle ear and mastoid. The degree of erosion depends on the size and location of the cholesteatoma. The main purpose of the tomographic study is therefore to determine the degree and extent of the pathology caused by the cholesteatoma.

When the cholesteatoma is limited to the middle ear cavity, the typical tomograph findings are erosion of the lateral epitympanic wall, erosion of the anterior tympanic spine, erosion of the posterosuperior canal wall, and erosion of the ossicular chain. As the cholesteatoma extends into the mastoid, the aditus becomes widened, the mastoid antrum enlarged and smooth in outline, and finally the trabecular pattern of the mastoid is destroyed with formation of a large cavity.

Two main radiographic patterns of cholesteatoma are observed depending upon the site of perforation. Cholesteatomas associated with a perforation of the pars flaccida are characterized by erosion of the anterior portion of the lateral wall of the epitympanum, destruction of the anterior tympanic spine, and extention of the soft tissue mass into the epitympanic recess lateral to the ossicles. The ossicles may be eroded and displaced medially. Cholesteatomas arising from a perforation of the pars tensa account for erosion of the posterior canal wall and of the posterior portion of the lateral wall of the epitympanum, destruction of the long process of the incus, and extention of the soft tissue mass into the epitympanic recess medial to the ossicles. In these cases the ossicles may be eroded and displaced laterally.

At times the cholesteatoma may erode the labyrinth. Labyrinthine fistulas usually involve the horizontal semicircular canal and are recognizable by the flattening of the convex bulge of the horizontal semicircular canal and by the destruction of the bony capsule surrounding the lumen of the canal.

The interpretation of the radiographic study performed after mastoidectomy is quite difficult. Following surgery several landmarks may be missing, and it is often impossible to determine whether the absence of these landmarks is due to the surgery, to destruction from the pathological process for which surgery was performed, or from recurrence of the cholesteatoma postoperatively.

In this atlas we will demonstrate six temporal bones with inflammation processes and cholesteatoma.

Acute and Subacute Otitis Media

There is evidence of acute and sub-acute otitis media in both temporal bones of this 22 month old child (Fig. 9.1–9.24) who died of congenital heart defects.

The right bone is sectioned in the coronal plane (Fig. 9.1–9.12) and the left in the sagittal plane (Fig. 9.13 to 9.24).

The first 2 mm thick coronal section of the right temporal bone crosses the external auditory canal, the epitympanum, the cochlea and the geniculate ganglion (Fig. 9.1–9.6.).

The mucosal lining of the middle ear and epitympanum is hypertrophic, thickened, and rugose. The narrowed lumen contains inspissated mucous.

In the tissue sections, the hypertrophic mucosa obscures the anatomical features.

The tomographs show the intact ossicles and a diffuse clouding of the middle ear. There is no bony erosion.

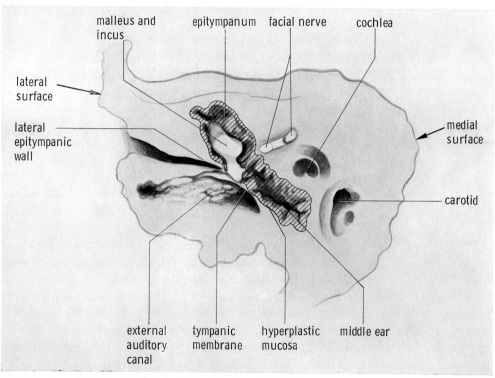

9.1   Drawing of structures and pathology seen in Fig. 9.2 to 9.6.

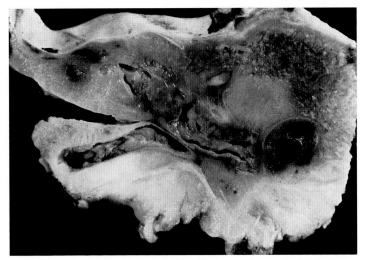

9.2   Photograph of anterior surface of a coronal macrosection at the level of the external auditory canal, epitympanum, and geniculate ganglion.

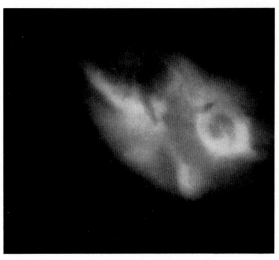

9.3   Tomograph corresponding to Fig. 9.2.

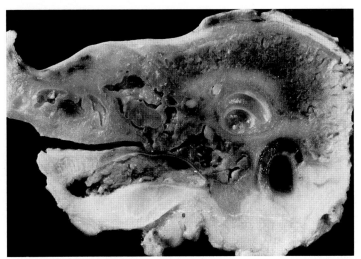

9.4   Photograph of posterior surface of coronal macrosection Fig. 9.2. Reversed photographically.

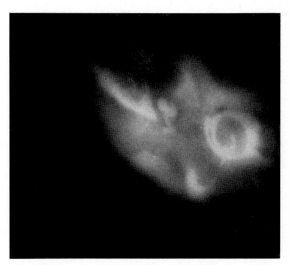

9.5   Tomograph corresponding to Fig. 9.4.

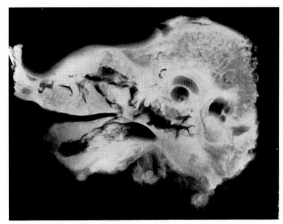

9.6   Microradiograph of coronal macrosection seen in Fig. 9.2 and 9.4.

Acute and Subacute Otitis Media

Figures 9.7–9.12 show acute and subacute otitis media in a 2 mm thick coronal section of the same right temporal bone 2 mm posterior to Fig. 9.1–9.6. The intervening 2 mm section has been omitted.

The section crosses the external auditory canal, the middle ear, the cochlea, the oval window, the horizontal and superior semicircular canals, the mastoid antrum, and the internal auditory canal.

Hyperplastic, hypertrophic mucosa lines the middle ear and atrum. There is inspissated mucous in the middle ear and antral lumina.

The tomographs show diffuse clouding of the middle ear and antrum without erosion of the ossicles or other bony structures.

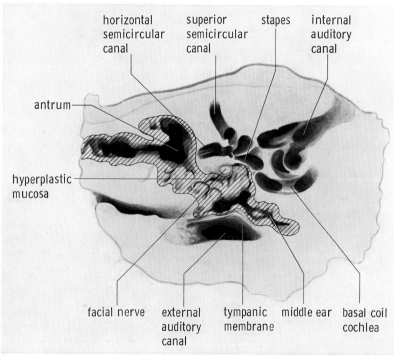

9.7   Drawing of structures and pathology seen in Fig. 9.8 to 9.12.

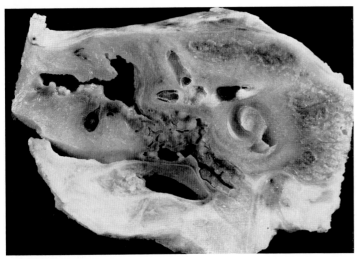

9.8   Photograph of anterior surface of the coronal macrosection 2 mm posterior to Fig. 9.4.

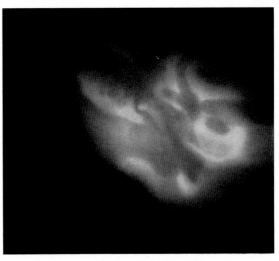

9.9   Tomograph corresponding to Fig. 9.8.

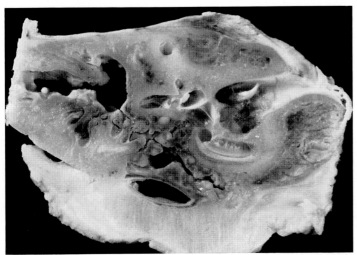

9.10   Photograph of posterior surface of coronal macrosection Fig. 9.8. Reversed photographically.

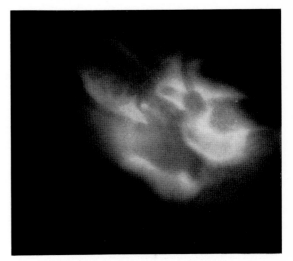

9.11   Tomograph corresponding to Fig. 9.10.

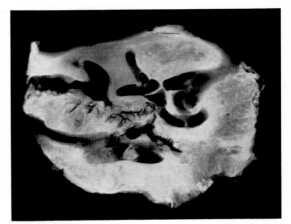

9.12   Microradiograph of coronal macrosection seen in Fig. 9.8 and 9.10.

Acute and Subacute Otitis Media

This left temporal bone is from the same patient as in Figs. 9.1–9.12. There is acute and sub-acute otitis media in these 2 mm thick sagittal sections of the left temporal bone (Fig. 9.13–9.24).

The first section crosses the external auditory canal, the middle ear, the tympanic membrane, the epitympanum, the antrum, and the descending portion of the facial nerve (Fig. 9.13–9.18).

The mucosa of the tympanic cavity, epitympanum, and antrum is hypertrophic, thickened, and rugose. The thickened mucosa obscures the portions of the malleus and incus present in the section.

The tomographs show diffuse cloudiness of the middle ear, epitympanum, antrum, and mastoid air cells. The ossicles are well visualized and intact.

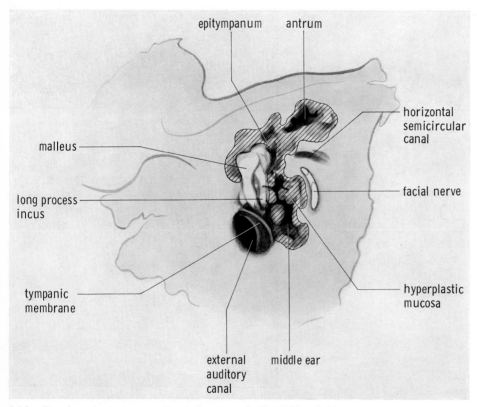

9.13   Drawing of structures and pathology seen in Fig. 9.14 to 9.18.

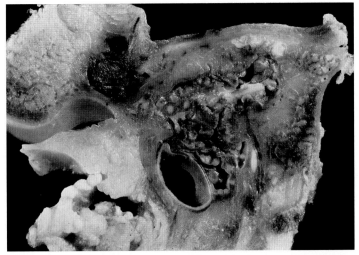

9.14   Photograph of lateral surface of a sagittal macrosection at the level of the external auditory canal, epitympanum, and mastoid antrum.

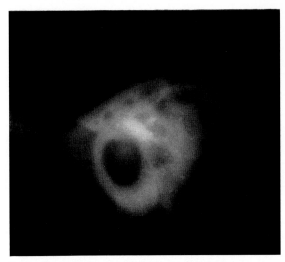

9.15   Tomograph corresponding to Fig. 9.14.

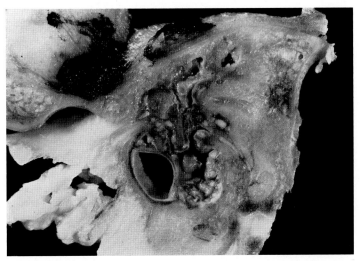

9.16   Photograph of medial surface of sagittal macrosection Fig. 9.14. Reversed photographically.

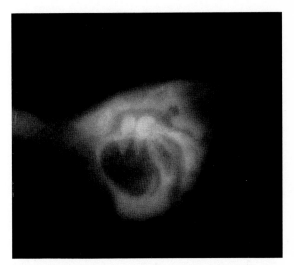

9.17   Tomograph corresponding to Fig. 9.16.

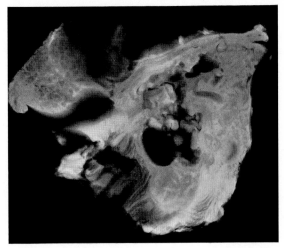

9.18   Microradiograph of sagittal macrosection seen in Fig. 9.14 and 9.16.

Acute and Subacute Otitis Media

Figures 9.19–9.24 show acute and sub-acute otitis media in a 2 mm thick sagittal section of the same left temporal bone immediately medial to Fig. 9.13–9.18. The section exposes the middle ear, the epitympanum, and the lateral and posterior semicircular canals.

The middle ear and antral mucosa is hypertrophic and rugose.
The tomographs show diffuse clouding of the lumen of the middle ear and mastoid air cells. The ossicles and other bony structures are intact.

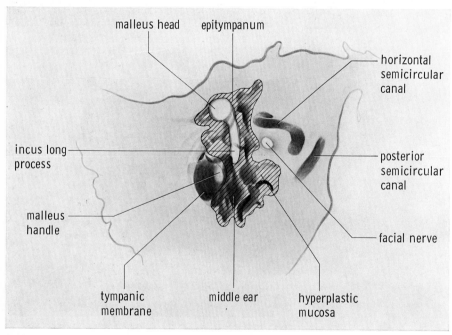

9.19   Drawing of structures and pathology seen in Fig. 9.20 to 9.24.

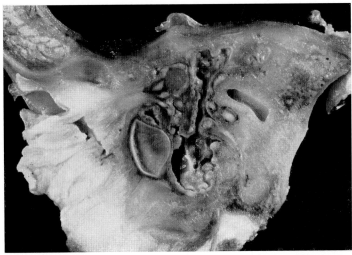

9.20   Photograph of lateral surface of the sagittal macrosection immediately medial to Fig. 9.16.

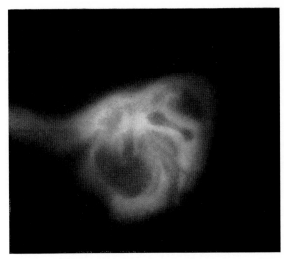

9.21   Tomograph corresponding to Fig. 9.20.

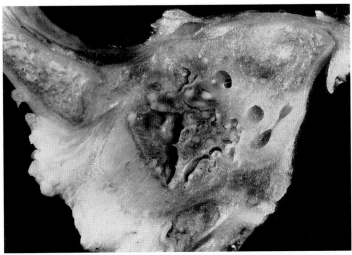

9.22   Photograph of medial surface of sagittal macrosection Fig. 9.20. Reversed photographically.

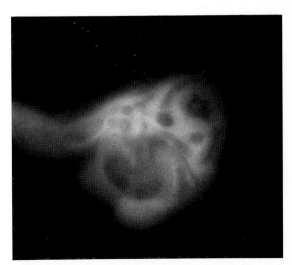

9.23   Tomograph corresponding to Fig. 9.22.

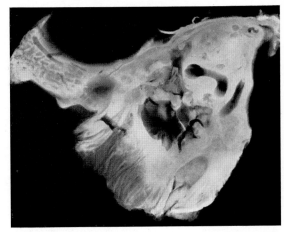

9.24   Microradiograph of sagittal macrosection seen in Fig. 9.20 and 9.21.

Chronic Otitis Media with Perforation of the Tympanic Membrane

In this temporal bone there was a chronic otitis media, and the tympanic membrane was perforated.

The sections of this right adult temporal bone (Fig. 9.25–9.53) are 2 mm thick and lie in the coronal plane. The first section exposes the external auditory canal, the anterior portion of the cochlea, the carotid artery, and the geniculate ganglion (Fig. 9.25–9.31).

The tympanic membrane is perforated, and a membranous fold stretches from the inferior margin of the perforation to the medial wall of the tympanic cavity.

The inflammatory process has eroded the inferior margin of the lateral epitympanic wall and the adjacent me-dial portion of the superior wall of the external auditory canal. In the tomographs this erosion accounts for the blunt appearance of the lateral epitympanic wall.

The epitympanum is filled with firm, fibrous, inflammatory tissue which surrounds the head of the malleus. Figure 9.53 shows the histopathology at this level. Figure 9.30 is a postmortem photograph of the tympanic membrane from the same right adult temporal bone with chronic otitis media (Fig. 9.25–9.53).

There is a large central type perforation of the pars tensa. Small nodules of chronic inflammatory tissue on the promontory are visible through the perforation.

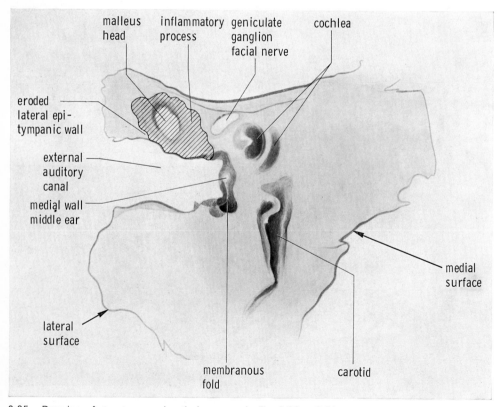

9.25   Drawing of structures and pathology seen in Fig. 9.26 to 9.31.

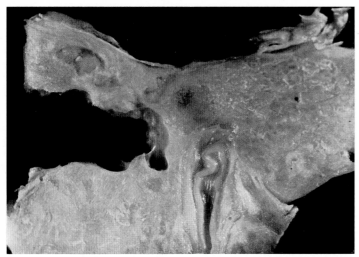

9.26   Photograph of anterior surface of a coronal macrosection at the level of the external auditory canal, the cochlea, and the carotid artery.

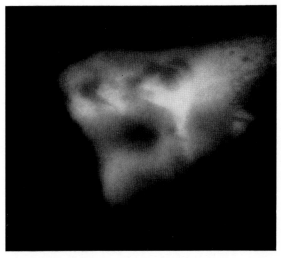

9.27   Tomograph corresponding to Fig. 9.26.

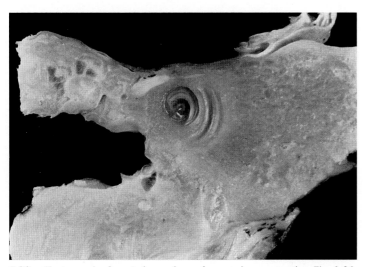

9.28   Photograph of posterior surface of coronal macrosection Fig. 9.26. Reversed photographically.

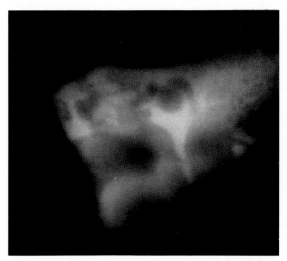

9.29   Tomograph corresponding to Fig. 9.28.

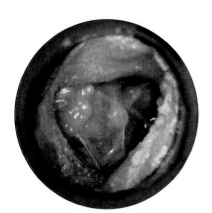

9.30   Tympanic membrane.

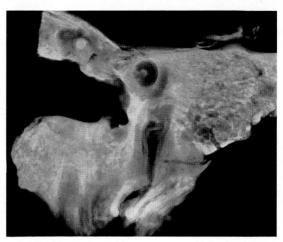

9.31   Microradiograph of coronal macrosection seen in Fig. 9.26 and 9.28.

Chronic Otitis Media with Perforation of the Tympanic Membrane

Figures 9.32–9.37 show the findings in a 2 mm thick coronal section of the same right adult temporal bone with chronic inflammatory disease immediately posterior to Fig. 9.25–9.31.

The section exposes the middle ear, the cochlea, and the geniculate ganglion.

The posterior margin of a central type tympanic membrane perforation lies between the middle and external ears.

The inferior margin of the lateral epitympanic wall is blunted, and fibrous, inflammatory tissue fills the epitympanum and surrounds the ossicles. This chronic inflammatory tissue obscures visualization of the ossicles in the macrosections (Fig. 9.26, 9.28, 9.33 and 9.35). In the tomographs, there is a soft tissue density in the attic surrounding the ossicles.

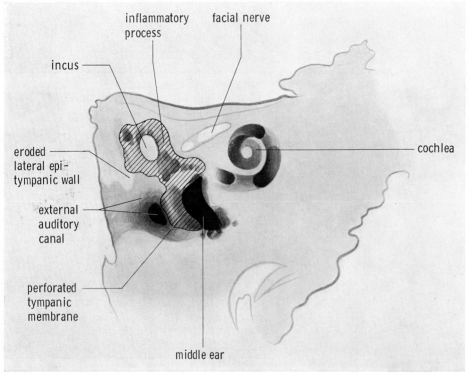

9.32   Drawing of structures and pathology seen in Fig. 9.33 to 9.37.

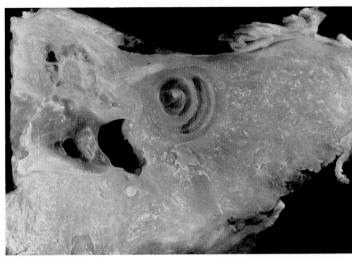

9.33 Photograph of anterior surface of a coronal macrosection immediately posterior to Fig. 9.28.

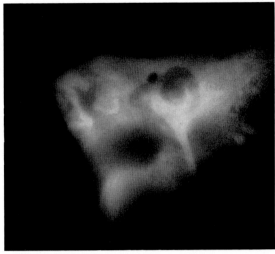

9.34 Tomograph corresponding to Fig. 9.33.

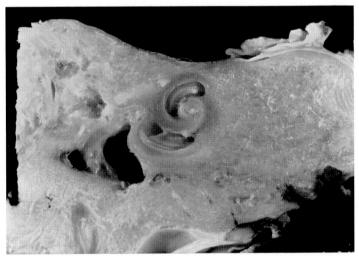

9.35 Photograph of posterior surface of coronal macrosection Fig. 9.33.
Reversed photographically.

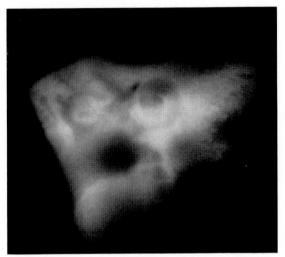

9.36 Tomograph corresponding to Fig. 9.35.

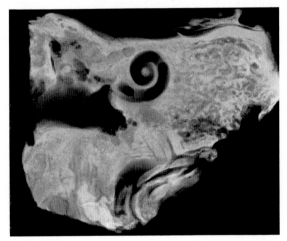

9.37 Microradiograph of coronal macrosection seen in
Fig. 9.33 and 9.35.

Chronic Otitis Media with Perforation of the Tympanic Membrane

Figures 9.38–9.43 show the pathology in a 2 mm thick coronal section of the same right adult temporal bone with chronic inflammatory disease immediately posterior to Fig. 9.32–9.37.

The section crosses the posterior portion of the middle ear, the vestibule, the basal turn of the cochlea, the superior and horizontal semicircular canal, and the internal auditory canal.

Fibrous inflammatory tissue fills the antrum and epitympanum and envelopes the stapes. The long process of the incus is eroded.

The tomographs show a soft tissue density in the epitympanum and upper tympanic cavity surrounding the eroded incus.

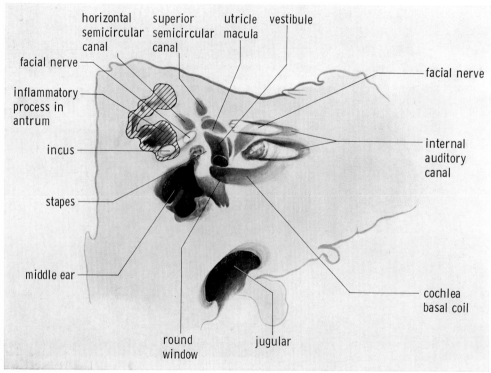

9.38   Drawing of structures and pathology seen in Fig. 9.39 to 9.43.

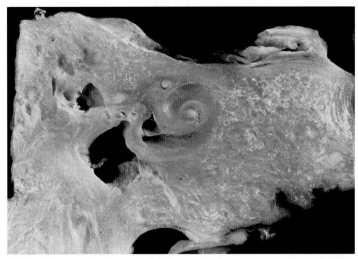

9.39 Photograph of anterior surface of a coronal macrosection immediately posterior to Fig. 9.35.

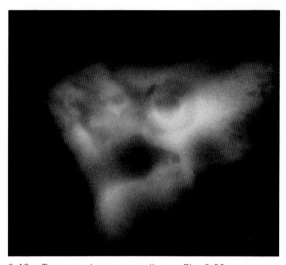

9.40 Tomograph corresponding to Fig. 9.39.

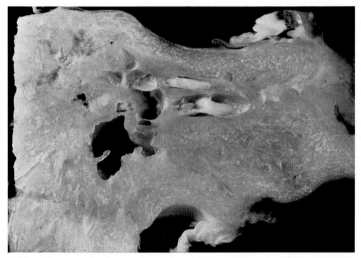

9.41 Photograph of posterior surface of coronal macrosection Fig. 9.39. Reversed photographically.

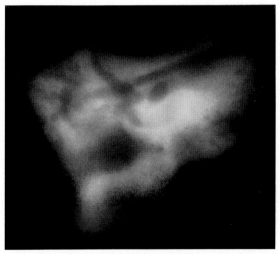

9.42 Tomograph corresponding to Fig. 9.41.

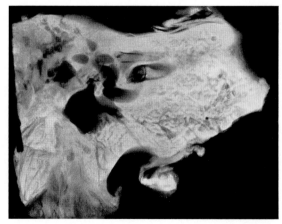

9.43 Microradiograph of coronal macrosection seen in Fig. 9.39 and 9.41.

Chronic Otitis Media with Perforation of the Tympanic Membrane

Figures 9.44–9.49 reveal the findings in a 2 mm thick coronal section of the same right adult temporal bone with chronic inflammatory disease immediately posterior to Fig. 9.38–9.43.
The section crosses the antrum, the superior and horizontal semicircular canals, the vestibule, and the internal auditory canal.
Firm fibrous tissue fills the small antrum. Thick, bony trabeculae narrow the lumen of the mastoid air cells. There is no bony erosion of the mastoid.

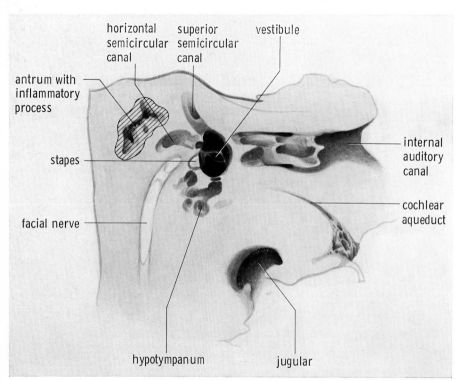

9.44   Drawing of structures and pathology seen in Fig. 9.45 to 9.49.

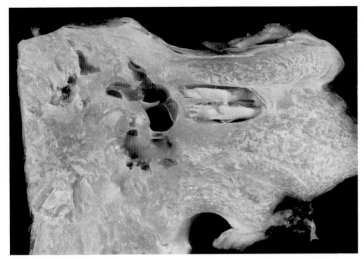

9.45   Photograph of anterior surface of a coronal macrosection immediately posterior to Fig. 9.41.

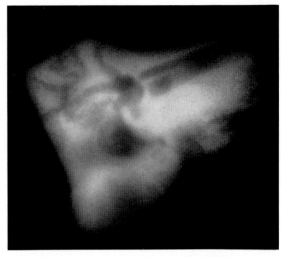

9.46   Tomograph corresponding to Fig. 9.45.

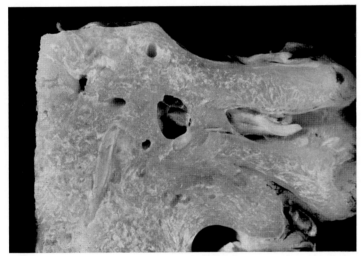

9.47   Photograph of posterior surface of coronal macrosection Fig. 9.45.
Reversed photographically.

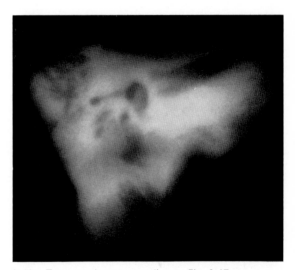

9.48   Tomograph corresponding to Fig. 9.47.

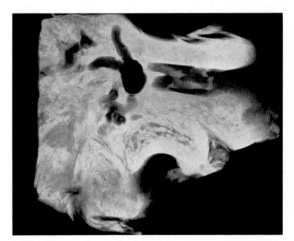

9.49   Microradiograph of coronal macrosection seen in
Fig. 9.45 and 9.47.

Chronic Otitis Media with Perforation of the Tympanic Membrane

These three sagittal tomographs (Fig. 9.50–9.52), 1 mm apart are from the same right adult temporal bone with chronic inflammatory disease as Fig. 9.25–9.53. The tomographs cross the epitympanum and show an intact anterior tympanic spine, malleus head, and incus body.

There is clouding of the posterior portion of the epitympanum extending to the posterosuperior quadrant of the tympanic cavity. The long process of the incus is eroded.

Histopathology Chronic Otitis Media with Perforation of the Tympanic Membrane

Figure 9.53 shows a low power photomicrograph of the macrosection in Fig. 9.26 and 9.28. The malleus head lies in the epitympanum surrounded by firm, fibrous, chronic inflammatory tissue. The lateral attic wall is eroded and calcified, tympanosclerotic tissue stretches from the lateral epitympanic wall to the medial wall of the epitympanum. Only a trace of the tympanic membrane is present inferiorly, and there are membranous folds in the hypotympanum.

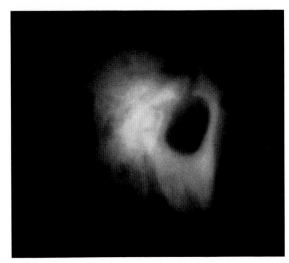

9.50   Sagittal tomograph.

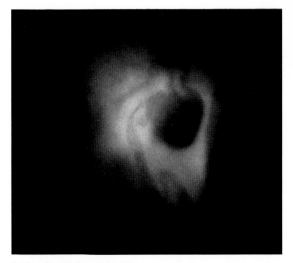

9.51   Sagittal tomograph.

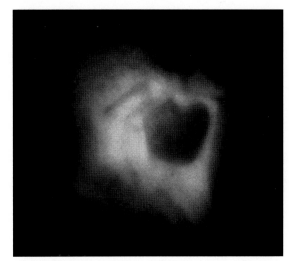

9.52   Sagittal tomograph.

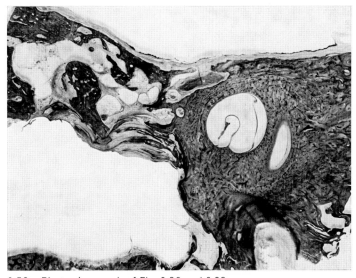

9.53   Photomicrograph of Fig. 9.26 and 9.28.

Chronic Otitis Media and Mastoiditis

Figures 9.54–9.80 demonstrate chronic otitis media and chronic mastoiditis.

The plane of the first 2 mm thick sagittal section of this left adult temporal bone (Fig. 9.54–9.59) lies at the level of the external auditory canal, the epitympanum, and the body of the incus.

The fibrous inflammatory tissue which fills the mastoid antrum and epitympanum surrounds and obscures the body of the incus.

The antrum is slightly enlarged and fairly smooth in outline due to some breakdown of the surrounding bony trabeculae.

The remainder of the mastoid shows diffuse thickening of the trabeculae and almost complete obliteration of the air cells.

There is slight erosion of the anterior aspect of the body of the incus. This erosion causes the anterior surface of the incus to have a concave rather than convex contour, Fig. 9.58 and 9.59.

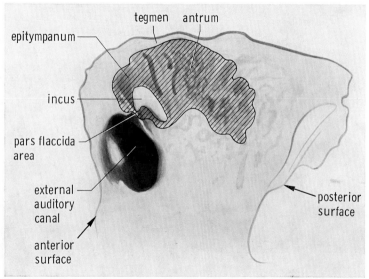

9.54 Drawing of structures and pathology seen in Fig. 9.55 to 9.59.

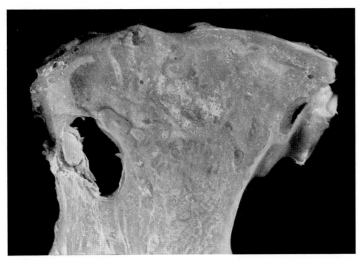

9.55 Photograph of lateral surface of a sagittal macrosection at the level of the epitympanum and external auditory canal.

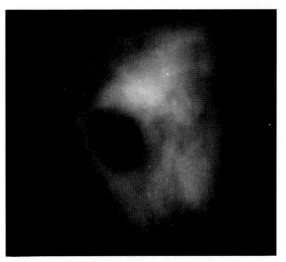

9.56 Tomograph corresponding to Fig. 9.55.

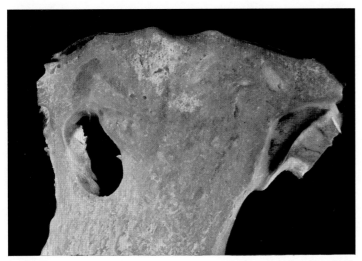

9.57 Photograph of medial surface of sagittal macrosection Fig. 9.55. Reversed photographically.

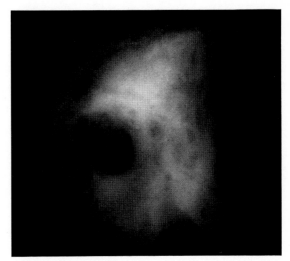

9.58 Tomograph corresponding to Fig. 9.57.

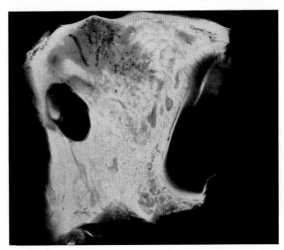

9.59 Microradiograph of sagittal macrosection seen in Fig. 9.55 and 9.57.

Chronic Otitis Media and Mastoiditis

Figures 9.60–9.65 show the findings in a left adult temporal bone with chronic otitis media and mastoiditis. This 2 mm thick sagittal section lies immediately medial to Fig. 9.54–9.59.

The section exposes the epitympanum, the antrum, the malleus head, and the body and short process of the incus.

The mastoid antrum is filled with chronic inflammatory tissue. There is tympanosclerosis in the epitympanum lying on the superior surface of the malleus head and incus body.

The anterior tympanic spine is normal. A few small globular cystic lesions with inspissated inflammatory exudate lie under the body of the incus.

The chorda tympani arches upward from the facial nerve.

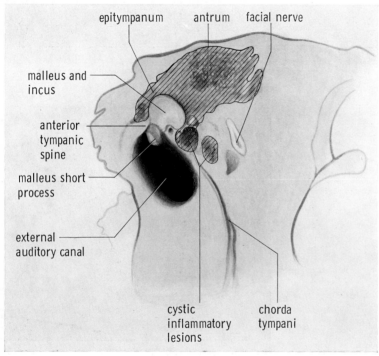

9.60 Drawing of structures and pathology seen in Fig. 9.61 to 9.65.

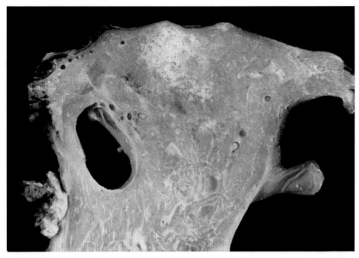

9.61 Photograph of lateral surface of a sagittal macrosection immediately medial to Fig. 9.57.

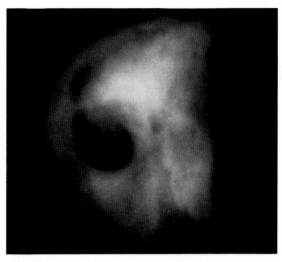

9.62 Tomograph corresponding to Fig. 9.61.

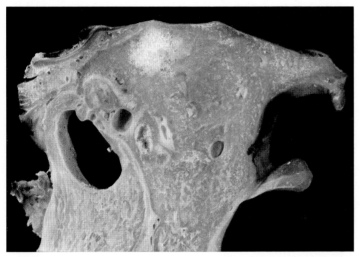

9.63 Photograph of medial surface of sagittal macrosection Fig. 9.61. Reversed photographically.

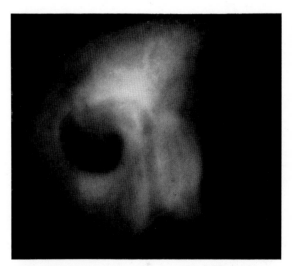

9.64 Tomograph corresponding to Fig. 9.63.

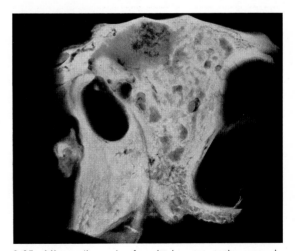

9.65 Microradiograph of sagittal macrosection seen in Fig. 9.61 and 9.63.

Chronic Otitis Media and Mastoiditis

Figures 9.66–9.71 demonstrate the findings in a left adult temporal bone with chronic otitis media and mastoiditis. This 2 mm thick sagittal section lies immediately medial to Fig. 9.60–9.65.

The section crosses the descending facial nerve and the epitympanum, and exposes the lateral arch of the horizontal semicircular canal.

Inflammatory debris fills the epitympanum. The anterior surface of the malleus head is eroded. There are cyst-like lesions in the middle ear medial to the thickened tympanic membrane.

The distal tip of the long process of the incus is eroded. This erosion is evident in the microradiograph (Fig. 9.71), and on the coronal tomographs (Fig. 9.78–9.80).

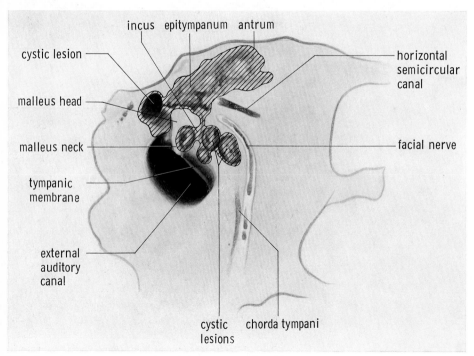

9.66 Drawing of structures and pathology seen in Fig. 9.67 to 9.71.

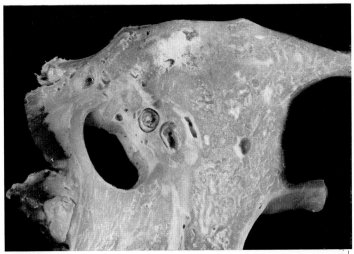

9.67 Photograph of lateral surface of a sagittal macrosection immediately medial to Fig. 9.63.

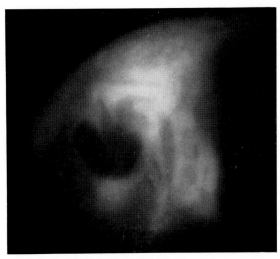

9.68 Tomograph corresponding to Fig. 9.67.

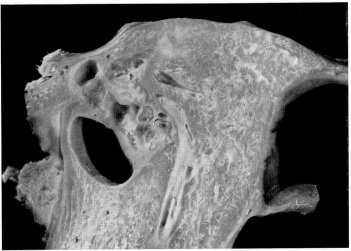

9.69   Photograph of medial surface of sagittal macrosection Fig. 9.67. Reversed photographically.

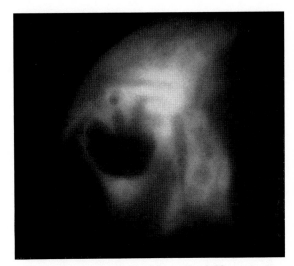

9.70 Tomograph corresponding to Fig. 9.69.

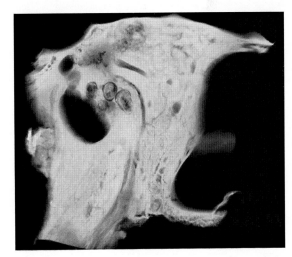

9.71   Microradiograph of sagittal macrosection seen in Fig. 9.67 and 9.69.

Chronic Otitis Media and Mastoiditis

Figures 9.72–9.77 show the findings in a left adult temporal bone with chronic otitis media and mastoiditis. This 2 mm thick sagittal section lies immediately medial to Fig. 9.66–9.71.
The section exposes the middle ear and the horizontal, superior, and posterior semicircular canals.

The thickened tympanic membrane separates the middle ear from the external auditory canal.
Thickened tympanosclerotic inflammatory tissue lies in the epitympanum and middle ear. Fibrous and tympanosclerotic tissue surround the stapes remnant.
In the tomographs, the middle ear appears cloudy.

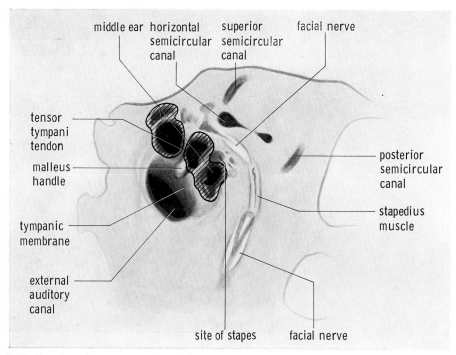

9.72 Drawing of structures and pathology seen in Fig. 9.73 to 9.77.

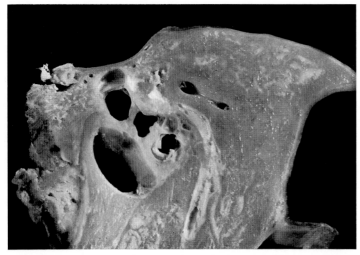

9.73 Photograph of lateral surface of a sagittal macrosection immediately medial to Fig. 9.69.

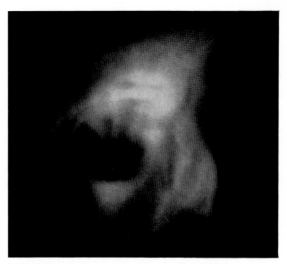

9.74 Tomograph corresponding to Fig. 9.73.

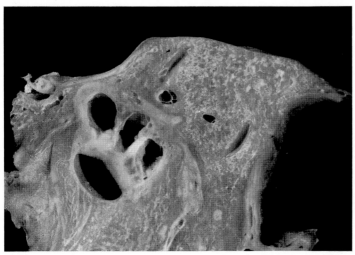

9.75 Photograph of medial surface of sagittal macrosection Fig. 9.73. Reversed photographically.

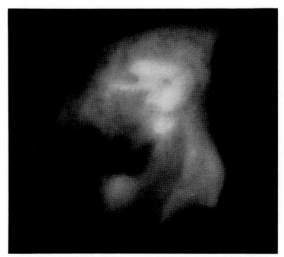

9.76 Tomograph corresponding to Fig. 9.75.

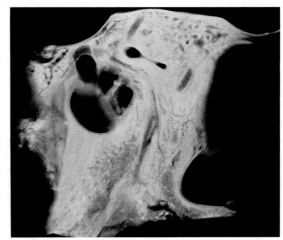

9.77 Microradiograph of sagittal macrosection seen in Fig. 9.73 and 9.75.

Chronic Otitis Media and Mastoiditis

Coronal tomographs (Fig. 9.78–9.80) of the same bone in Fig. 9.54–9.77 reveal some interesting features of chronic otitis media and mastoiditis.

The first tomograph crosses at the level of the cochlea (Fig. 9.78). The second section lies 3 mm posterior (Fig. 9.79). The third section crosses the antrum (Fig. 9.80).

The lateral wall of the epitympanum is intact. The tympanic membrane is thickened and a soft tissue density fills the antrum, epitympanum, and upper mesotympanum.

The ossicles appear normal except for the absence of the distal tip of the long process of the incus.

In these sections the tomographs do not show any of the typical radiographic features of cholesteatoma.

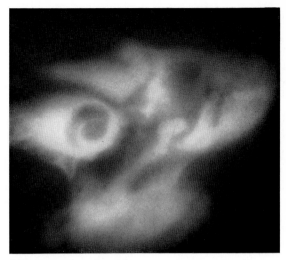

9.78 Coronal tomograph

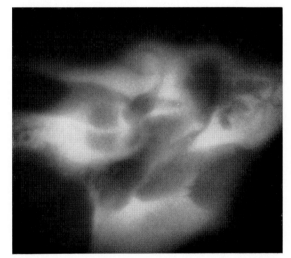

9.79 Coronal tomograph

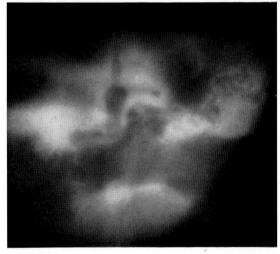

9.80 Coronal tomograph

Cholesteatoma, Small Epitympanic Type

In this left adult temporal bone there is a small, epitympanic cholesteatoma arising from the pars flaccida of the tympanic membrane (Fig. 9.81–9.114). There is no epithelial debris within the lumen of the cholesteatoma sac. The sections are in the sagittal plane and each section is 2 mm thick.

The first section lies at the level of the mastoid antrum and exposes the lateral portion of the epitympanum, (Fig. 9.81–9.86).

A small portion of the wall of the cholesteatoma sac appears on the medial surface of the section in the ante-

rior and lateral portion of the epitympanum, (Fig. 9.84). The short process of the incus rests in the fossa incudis. The antrum is large and well aerated. The outline is intact, but smooth. In small mastoids such as this, the antrum often has the appearance of a single, large, smooth, air-filled cavity. This appearance is due to the absence of surrounding air cells and trabeculae which give the antrum its usual scalloped outline.

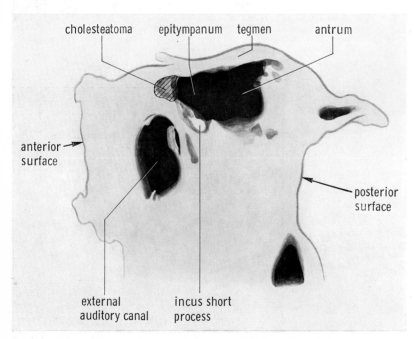

9.81   Drawing of structures and pathology seen in Fig. 9.82 to 9.86.

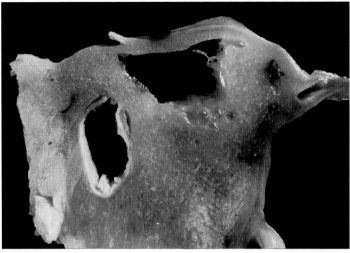

9.82 Photograph of lateral surface of a sagittal macrosection at the level of the epitympanum and antrum.

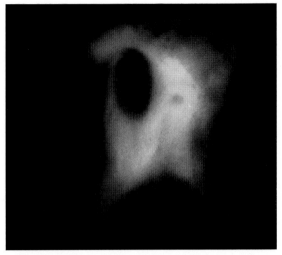

9.83 Tomograph corresponding to Fig. 9.82.

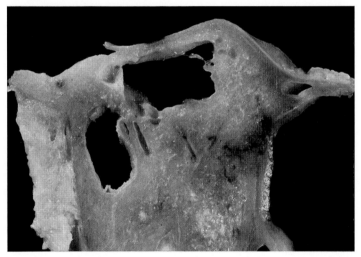

9.84 Photograph of medial surface of sagittal macrosection Fig. 9.82. Reversed photographically.

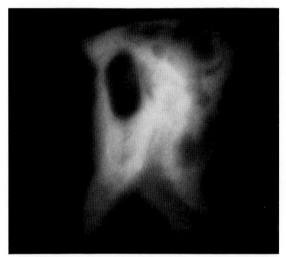

9.85 Tomograph corresponding to Fig. 9.84.

9.86. Microradiograph of sagittal macrosection seen in Fig. 9.82 and 9.89.

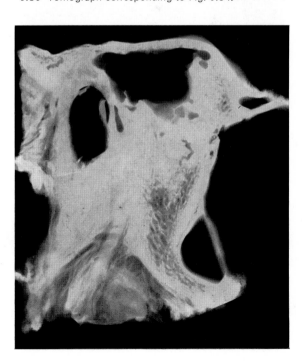

Cholesteatoma, Small Epitympanic Type

Figures 9.87–9.93 show a small epitympanic cholesteatoma in a 2 mm thick sagittal section of the same left adult temporal bone immediately medial to Fig. 9.81 to 9.86.

The section exposes the perforation in the pars flaccida region of the tympanic membrane, a portion of the incus, and the descending facial nerve.

The epitympanic perforation occupies the superior portion of the external auditory canal. The section demonstrates the entire circumference of the cholesteatoma sac. The sac extends superiorly from the posterior margin of the perforation, lies in contact with the anterior aspect of the incus body, covers the tegmen, extends along the anterior wall of the epitympanum, and erodes the anterior tympanic spine.

The remaining epitympanum and antrum are free of disease.

See Fig. 9.113 for the histopathology of this section. Figure 9.92 is a postmortem photograph of the tympanic membrane taken from the same left adult temporal bone with an epitympanic cholesteatoma as Fig. 9.81 to 9.114.

There is a perforation characteristic of epitympanic cholesteatomas in the pars flaccida region above the malleus short process.

The pars tensa is intact and the malleus handle extends inferior from the short process.

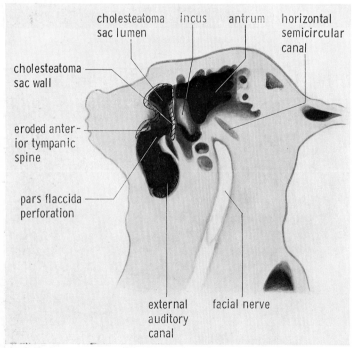

9.87 Drawing of structures and pathology seen in Fig. 9.88 to 9.93.

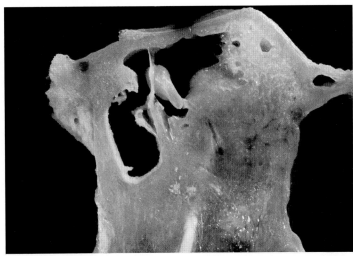

9.88 Photograph of lateral surface of a sagittal macrosection immediately medial to Fig. 9.84.

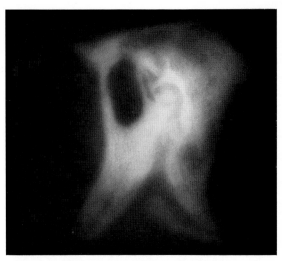

9.89 Tomograph corresponding to Fig. 9.88.

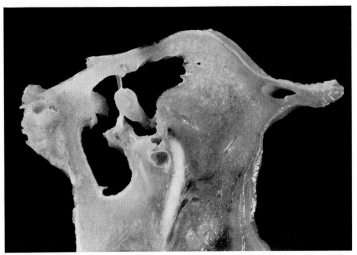

9.90 Photograph of medial surface of sagittal macrosection Fig. 9.88. Reversed photographically.

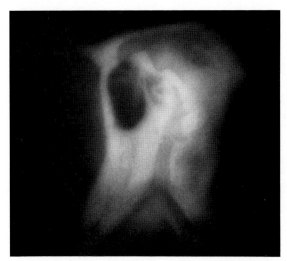

9.91 Tomograph corresponding to Fig. 9.90.

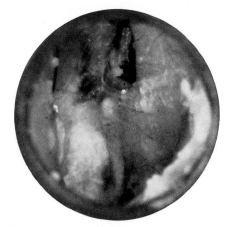

9.92 Tympanic membrane.

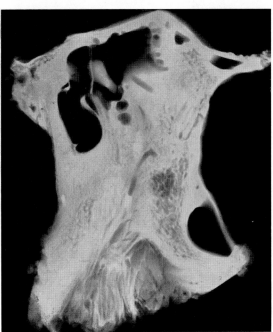

9.93 Microradiograph of sagittal macrosection seen in Fig. 9.88 and 9.90.

Cholesteatoma, Small Epitympanic Type

Figures 9.94–9.99 show a small, attic epitympanic cholesteatoma in a 2 mm thick sagittal section of the same left adult temporal bone immediately medial to Fig. 9.87–9.93.

The section crosses the ossicles in the epitympanum and the horizontal and posterior semicircular canals.

The medial portion of the cholesteatoma sac extends from the pars flaccida perforation to the tegmen. The sac lines the anterior wall of the epitympanum and erodes the anterior portion of the malleus head.

The remaining structures in the epitympanum and middle ear are normal.

The chorda tympani stretches across the middle ear lateral to the long process of the incus.

See Fig. 9.114 for the histopathology of this section.

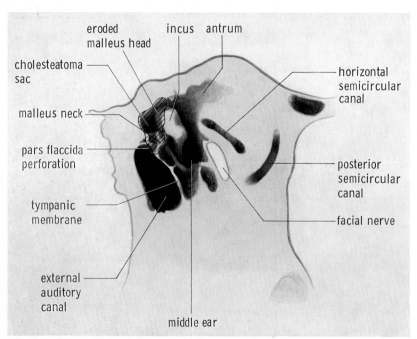

9.94 Drawing of structures and pathology seen in Fig. 9.95 zo 9.99.

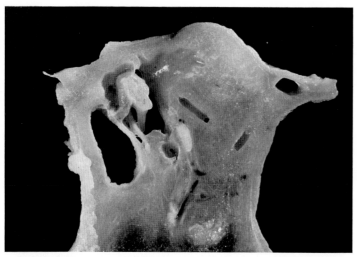

9.95 Photograph of lateral surface of a sagittal macrosection immediately medial to Fig. 9.90.

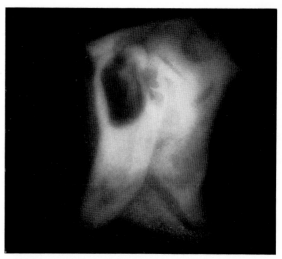

9.96 Tomograph corresponding to Fig. 9.95.

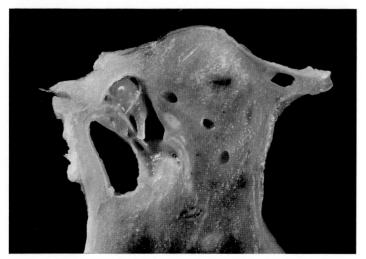

9.97 Photograph of medial surface of sagittal macrosection Fig. 9.95. Reversed photographically.

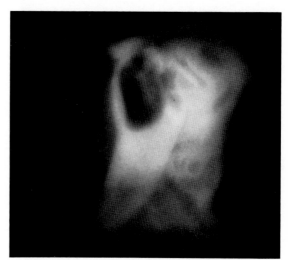

9.98 Tomograph corresponding to Fig. 9.97.

9.99 Microradiograph of sagittal macrosection seen in Fig. 9.95 and 9.97.

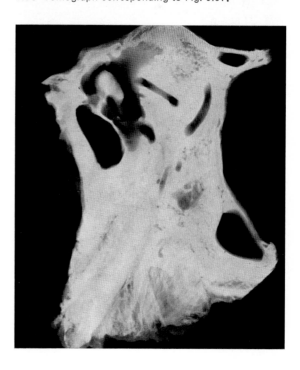

Cholesteatoma, Small Epitympanic Type

Figures 9.100–9.105 show the findings in a 2 mm thick sagittal section of the same left adult temporal bone with a small epitympanic cholesteatoma immediately medial to Fig. 9.94–9.99.

The section lies at the level of the stapes and cochleari-form process. The tympanic membrane is thickened, but all other structures are normal. There is no extension of the cholesteatoma.

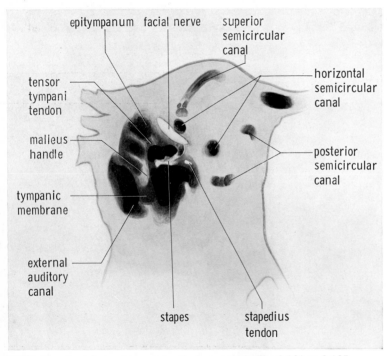

9.100 Drawing of structures and pathology seen in Fig. 9.101 to 9.105.

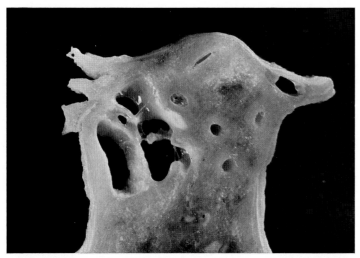

9.101 Photograph of lateral surface of a sagittal macrosection immediately medial to Fig. 9.97.

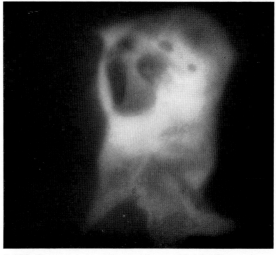

9.102 Tomograph corresponding to Fig. 9.101.

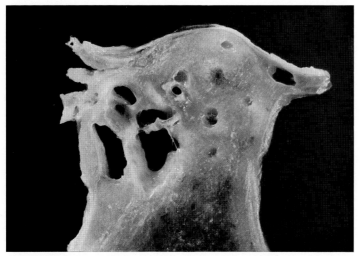

9.103 Photograph of medial surface of sagittal macrosection Fig. 9.101. Reversed photographically.

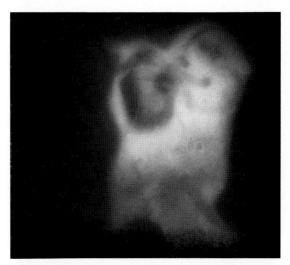

9.104 Tomograph corresponding to Fig. 9.103.

9.105 Microradiograph of sagittal macrosection seen in Fig. 9.101 and 9.103.

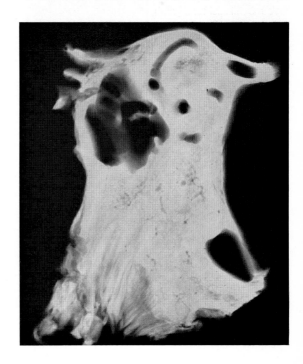

Cholesteatoma, Small Epitympanic Type

These three consecutive semiaxial tomographs (Fig. 106–108), 1 mm apart, are from the same left adult temporal bone with a small epitympanic cholesteatoma as Fig. 9.81–9.114.

These sections demonstrate the erosion of the inferior margin of the lateral epitympanic wall and thickening of the anterior portion of the tympanic membrane.

The remaining structures of the ear are normal. Fig. 9.108 clearly demonstrates the normal superstructure of the stapes.

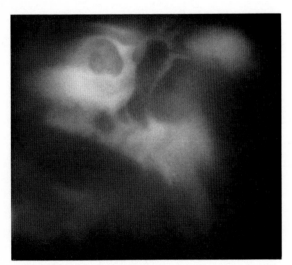

9.106 Semiaxial tomograph

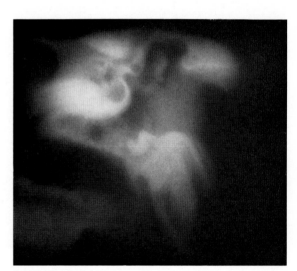

9.107 Semiaxial tomograph

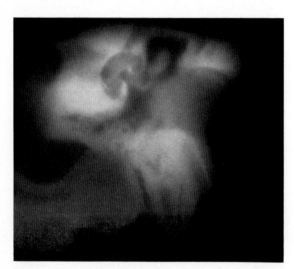

9.108 Semiaxial tomograph

Cholesteatoma, Small Epitympanic Type

These four consecutive coronal tomographic sections (Fig. 9.109–9.112), 1 mm apart, are from the same left adult temporal bone with a small epitympanic cholesteatoma as in Fig. 9.81–9.114.

A soft tissue mass erodes the inferior margin of the lateral epitympanic wall and the adjacent medial portion of the superior wall of the external auditory canal. The mass extends lateral to the malleus head, and the lateral aspect of the malleus head is slightly eroded.

The tympanic membrane is thicker and denser than normal.

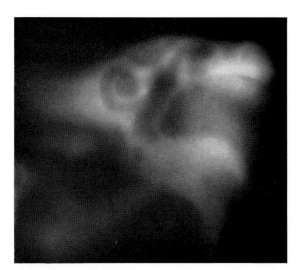

9.109 Coronal tomograph

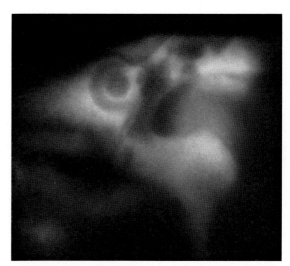

9.110 Coronal tomograph

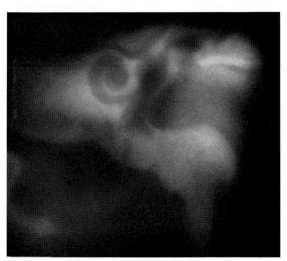

9.111 Coronal tomograph

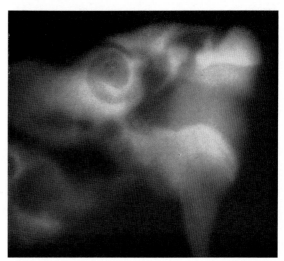

9.112 Coronal tomograph

Cholesteatoma, Small Epitympanic Type

Figure 9.113 is a low-power photomicrograph of the macrosection in Fig. 9.88 and 9.90.

The thin cholesteatoma matrix extends into the epitympanum from the pars flaccida perforation. The matrix lies in contact with the body of the incus, extends upward to the tegmen and lines the anterior portion of the epitympanum.

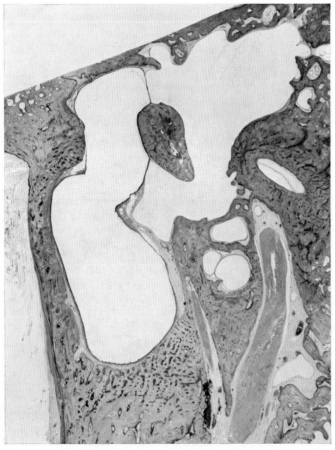

9.113 Photomicrograph of Fig. 9.88 and 9.90.

Cholesteatoma, Small Epitympanic Type

Figure 9.114 is a low power photomicrograph of the macrosection in Fig. 9.95 and 9.97.

The cholesteatoma matrix appears as a thin-walled ring of stratified squamous epithelium in the anterior epitympanum. The cyst lies between the malleus head and the anterior wall of the epitymanum.

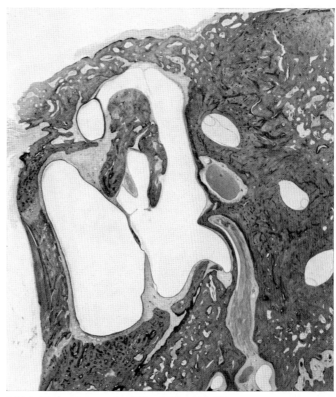

9.114 Photomicrograph of Fig. 9.95 and 9.97.

Cholesteatoma, Post Mastoidectomy

This adult temporal bone shows the findings following a modified radical mastoidectomy (Fig. 9.115–9.132). The surgery was performed for cholesteatoma several years before death.

The sections of this right bone lie in the coronal plane. Each tissue section is 2 mm thick.

The anterior surface of the first section (Fig. 9.115–9.120) exposes the anterior margin of the cochlea, the anterior middle ear, the geniculate ganglion, and the carotid artery.

Cholesteatoma debris and matrix fill the epitympanum, surround the malleus head, and extend into the lateral portion of the mesotympanum. In the tomographs, a soft tissue mass fills the epitympanum and upper mesotympanum.

Adhesive bands cross the middle ear.

There is erosion of the lateral epitympanic wall and of the lateral surface of the malleus head. The tomographs show the increased distance between the lateral epitympanic wall and the malleus head due to this erosion.

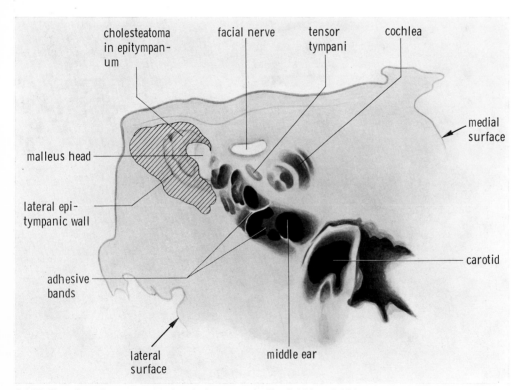

9.115 Drawing of structures and pathology seen in Fig. 9.116 to 9.120.

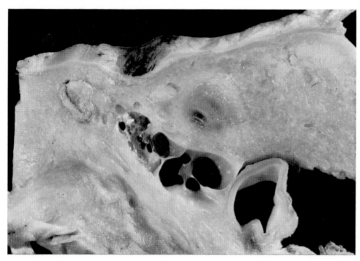

9.116 Photograph of anterior surface of a coronal macrosecretion at the level of anterior portion of the cochlea and anterior middle ear.

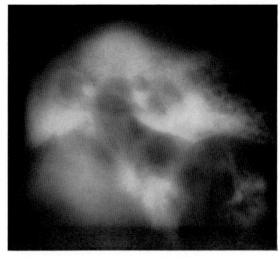

9.117 Tomograph corresponding to Fig. 9.116.

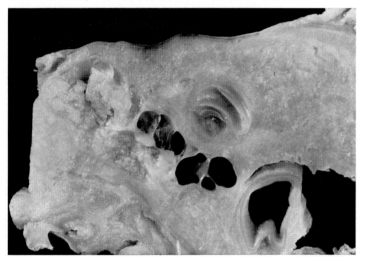

9.118 Photograph of posterior surface of coronal macrosection Fig. 9.116. Reversed photographically.

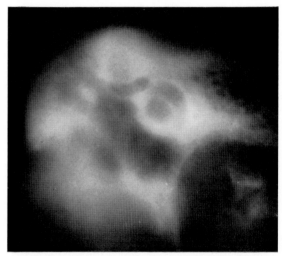

9.119 Tomograph corresponding to Fig. 9.118.

9.120 Microradiograph of coronal macrosection seen in Fig. 9.116 and 9.118.

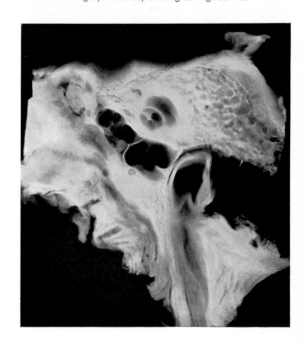

Cholesteatoma, Post Mastoidectomy

Figures 9.121–9.126 show the post mastoidectomy findings, in a 2 mm thick coronal section of the same right adult temporal bone posterior to Fig. 9.115–9.120.

A 2 mm thick section of bone between this section and Fig. 9.118, has been omitted.

The section crosses the external auditory canal, the middle ear, the vestibule, the superior semicircular canal, the facial nerve, and the internal auditory canal.

The surgical procedure created a mastoidectomy cavity by removing the posterior and superior walls of the external auditory canal and the adjacent lateral epitympanic wall.

Cholesteatoma matrix lines the entire mastoidectomy cavity from the tegmen tympani to the floor of the middle ear.

There is a stenosis of the external auditory canal laterally.

In the tomographs, a large soft tissue mass surrounds the eroded body of the incus and fills the surgical mastoid cavity and upper portion of the middle ear.

The soft tissue mass consisted of necrotic epithelial debris, but the mass and incus remnant disintegrated during the sectioning of the bone.

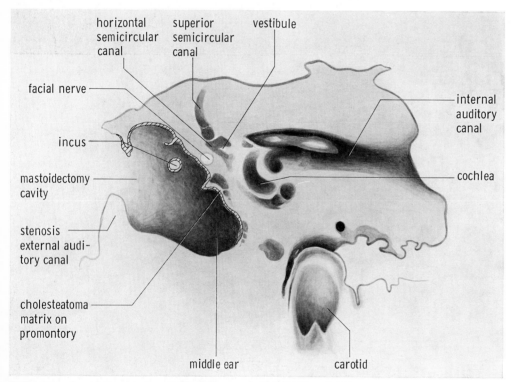

9.121   Drawing of structures and pathology seen in Fig. 9.122 to 9.126.

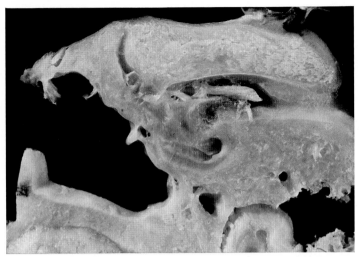

9.122 Photograph of anterior surface of a coronal macrosection 2 mm posterior to Fig. 9.118.

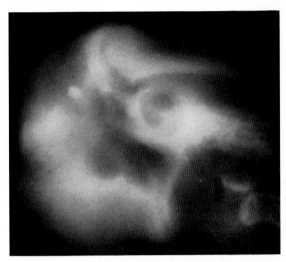

9.123 Tomograph corresponding to Fig. 9.122.

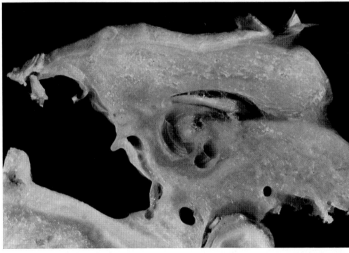

9.124 Photograph of posterior surface of coronal macrosection Fig. 9.122. Reversed photographically.

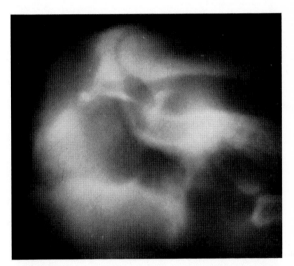

9.125 Tomograph corresponding to Fig. 9.124.

9.126 Microradiograph of coronal macrosection seen in Fig. 9.122 and 9.124.

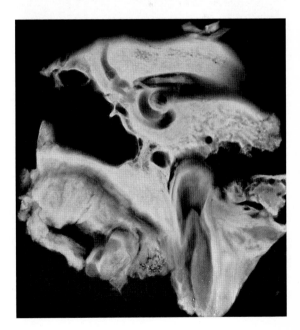

Cholesteatoma, Post Mastoidectomy

Figures 9.127–9.132 demonstrate the post mastoidectomy findings in a 2 mm thick coronal section of the same right adult temporal bone posterior to Fig. 9.121–9.126. A 2 mm thick section of bone between this section and Fig. 9.124, has been omitted.

This section reveals the horizontal and superior semicircular canals, the vestibule, the basal turn of the cochlea, and the posterior wall of the internal auditory canal.

The enlarged mastoid antrum is the result of the mastoidectomy. Cholesteatoma matrix lines the enlarged surgical cavity.

There is a large mass of epithelial debris in the posterior portion of the middle ear below the horizontal semicircular canal.

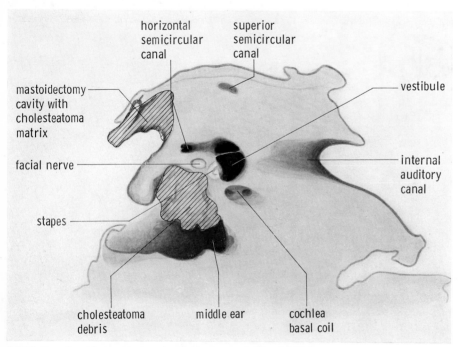

9.127 Drawing of structures and pathology seen in Fig. 9.128 to 9.132.

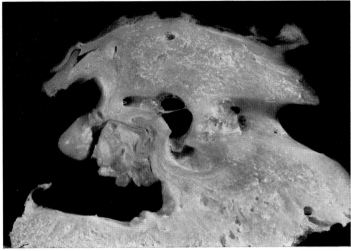

9.128 Photograph of anterior surface of a coronal macrosection 2 mm posterior to Fig. 9.124.

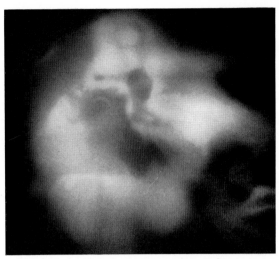

9.129 Tomograph corresponding to Fig. 9.128.

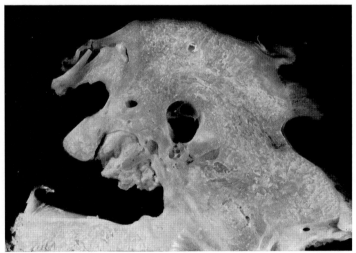

9.130 Photograph of posterior surface of coronal macrosection Fig. 9.128. Reversed photographically.

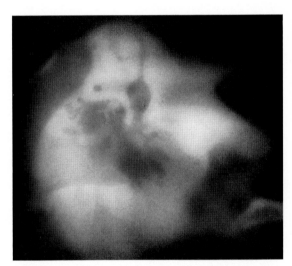

9.131 Tomograph corresponding to Fig. 9.130.

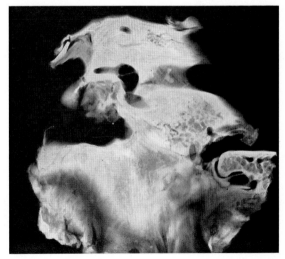

9.132 Microradiograph of coronal macrosection seen in Fig. 9.128 and 9.130.

Chapter 10 Otosclerosis

Tomography is the only radiographic method to study the labyrinthine windows and the labyrinthine capsule. We routinely use coronal and semiaxial sections of both petrous pyramids, 1 mm apart. The axial projection is also helpful.

In the coronal and semiaxial sections, the normal oval window appears as a well-defined bony dehiscence in the inferolateral wall of the vestibule below the opening of the horizontal semicircular canal. The normal footplate of the stapes is too thin to cast a definite line.

In fenestral otosclerosis, the anterior contour of the oval window usually becomes poorly defined. As the process progresses, there is narrowing or complete obliteration of the oval window by a bony plate of variable thickness and density.

Otosclerosis involving the cochlea produces a more or less severe disruption of the cochlear capsule. The normal capsule appears as a sharply defined, homogenously dense bony shell outlining the lumen of the cochlea.

The radiographic changes of cochlear otosclerosis vary upon the extent and type of involvement. The type of involvement depends upon the maturation of the pathological process. Actively enlarging, vascular otosclerotic foci appear as areas of demineralization in the cochlear bone. Sclerotic changes are the result of mature or maturing foci, and they are formed by the apposition of mature otosclerotic bone to the otic capsule. In the tomographs, these sclerotic foci, when seen in pro-

file, appear as areas of capsular thickening producing roughening or scalloping of the outer and inner aspects of the otic capsule. When seen face on, these sclerotic changes appear as areas of increased density superimposed upon the radiolucency of the cochlear lumen.

The usefullness of tomography in otosclerosis can be summarized as follows:

1) Diagnosis. There are cases in which otosclerosis cannot be diagnosed clinically with certainty, especially in cases of severe mixed deafness in which bone conduction is markedly depressed;

2) Evaluation of the extent and type of involvement of the oval window. In some cases tomographic evaluation may be useful in selecting the side for corrective surgery;

3) Evaluation of the post surgical status. Tomography is helpful in determining the position of radioopaque prostheses and in visualizing possible reobliteration of the oval window;

4) Demonstration of foci of labyrinthine otosclerosis in patients with clinical otosclerosis and in some patients with pure sensorineural hearing loss. Foci of otosclerosis in the cochlea and in other areas of the otic capsule, 2 mm in diameter and larger, can be demonstrated tomographically.

In this atlas we will demonstrate the findings in one temporal bone affected with otosclerosis.

Otosclerosis, Post-Stapedectomy

This 51-year-old man died suddenly from a massive intracranial hemorrhage.

In each ear there was evidence of otosclerosis and a previous stapedectomy. The illustrations (Fig. 10.1 to 10.20) demonstrate the findings in the right temporal bone.

The following 2 mm thick sections lie in the semiaxial plane. Figures 10.1–10.6 expose the external canal, the middle ear, the cochlea, and the internal auditory canal. On the posterior surface of the section there is an otosclerotic focus in the otic capsule at the anterior margin of the oval window. This focus extends to the upper margin of the scala vestibuli (Fig. 10.4).

A cleft at the anterior margin of the oval window appears to divide the focus into two lobules. This otosclerotic focus appears in the tomograph (Fig. 10.5). See Fig. 10.20 for the histopathology of this section. The malleus handle is attached to a strip of tympanic membrane. The tendon of the tensor tympani passes from the cochleariform process to the malleus neck, and a portion of the malleus head is in the epitympanum. The facial nerve lies above the tensor tympani muscle and the cochleariform process.

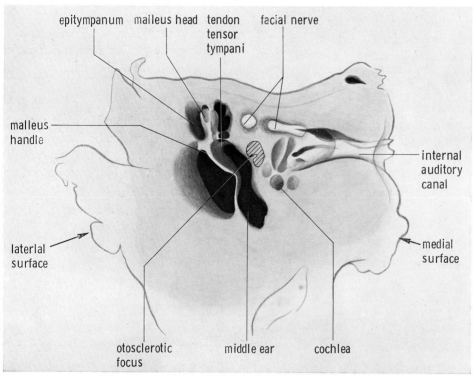

10.1   Drawing of structures and pathology seen in Fig. 10.2 to 10.6.

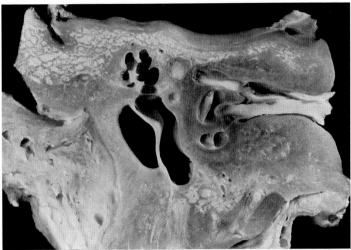

10.2   Photograph of anterior surface of a semiaxial macrosection at the level of the external auditory canal, the cochlea, and the internal auditory canal.

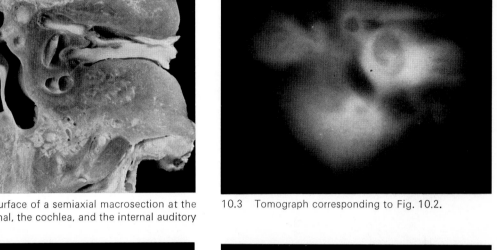

10.3   Tomograph corresponding to Fig. 10.2.

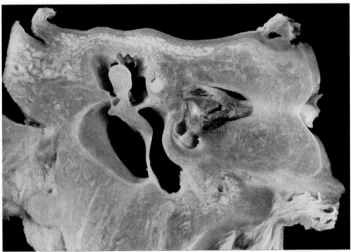

10.4   Photograph of posterior surface of semiaxial macrosection Fig. 10.2. Reversed photographically.

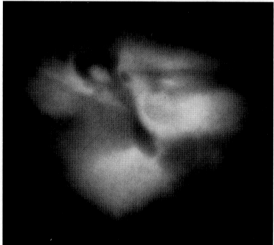

10.5   Tomograph corresponding to Fig. 10.4.

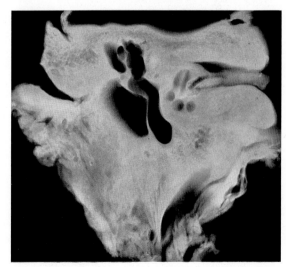

10.6   Microradiograph of semiaxial macrosection seen in Fig. 10.2 and 10.4.

Otosclerosis, Post-Stapedectomy

Fig. 10.7–10.12 reveal the findings in a 2 mm thick semi-axial section of the same right adult temporal bone with otosclerosis, immediately posterior to Figs. 10.1 to 10.6.

The section shows the external canal, the middle ear, and the fundus of the internal auditory canal.

A wire stapes prosthesis is attached to the long process of the incus and ends in a loop in the oval window.

On the anterior surface of the section (Fig. 10.8) the otosclerotic focus narrows the anterior margin of the oval window.

A section of the malleus head, incus body, and anterior half of the bisected long process of the incus are present. On the posterior surface of section (Fig. 10.10) the loop at the vestibular end of the wire prosthesis is imbedded in the fibrous tissue which fills the oval window.

In the tomographs, the wire prosthesis appears as a thin radioopaque line from the long process of the incus to the oval window area. The oval window is narrowed but patent in its central portion.

The round window appears on the posterior surface of the section.

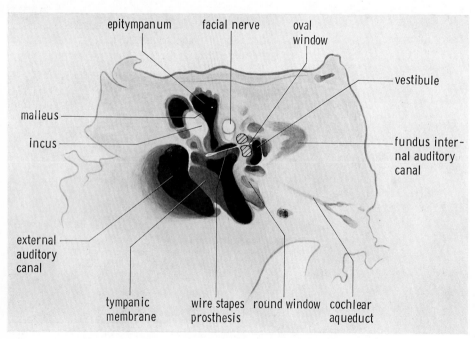

10.7   Drawing of structures and pathology seen in Fig. 10.8 to 10.12.

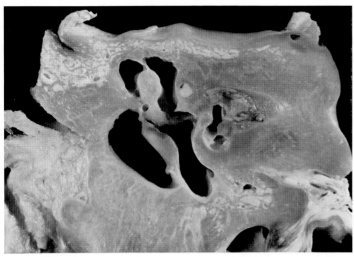

10.8 Photograph of anterior surface of the semiaxial macrosection immediately posterior to Fig. 10.4.

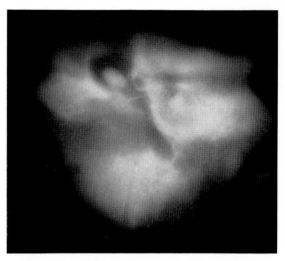

10.9 Tomograph corresponding to Fig. 10.8.

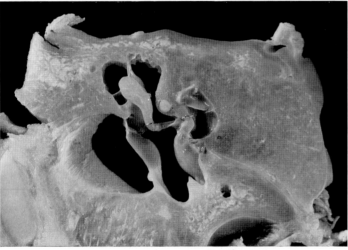

10.10 Photograph of posterior surface of semiaxial macrosection Fig. 10.8. Reversed photographically.

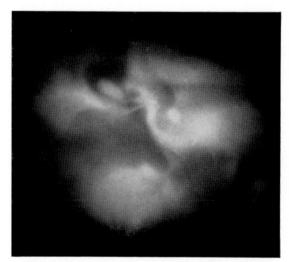

10.11 Tomograph corresponding to Fig. 10.10.

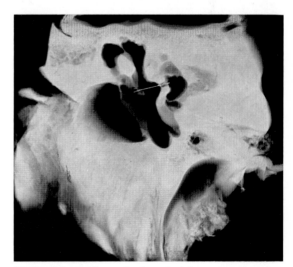

10.12 Microradiograph of semiaxial macrosection seen in Fig. 10.8 and 10.10.

Otosclerosis, Post-Stapedectomy

Figures 10.13–10.18 show the findings in a 2 mm thick semi-axial section of the same right adult temporal bone with otosclerosis immediately posterior to Fig. 10.7 to 10.12.

The section exposes the external auditory canal, the middle ear, and the horizontal and superior semicircular canals.

On the anterior surface of the section the otosclerotic focus involves the posterior portion of the oval window and extends into the promontory above the uninvolved round window (Fig. 10.14).

See Fig. 10.21 for the histopathology of this section.

The long process of the incus is sectioned longitudinally.

Portions of the membranous labyrinth are present, and the macula of the utricle stretches across the upper portion of the vestibule in close relation to oval window and otosclerotic focus.

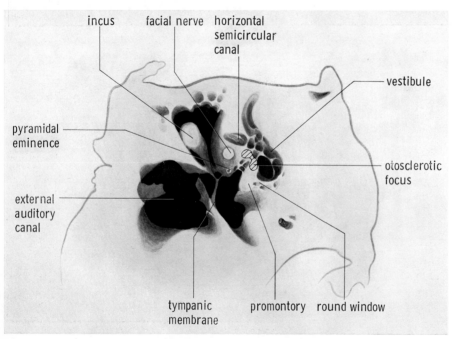

10.13   Drawing of structures and pathology seen in Fig. 10.14 to 10.18.

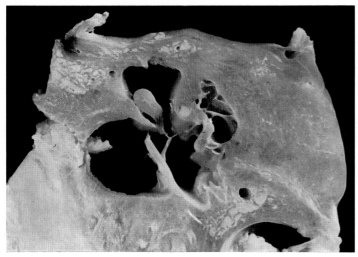

10.14   Photograph of anterior surface of the semiaxial macrosection immediately posterior to Fig. 10.10.

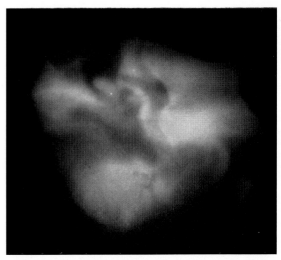

10.15   Tomograph corresponding to Fig. 10.14.

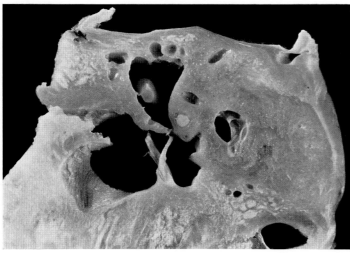

10.16   Photograph of posterior surface of semiaxial macrosection Fig. 10.14. Reversed photographically.

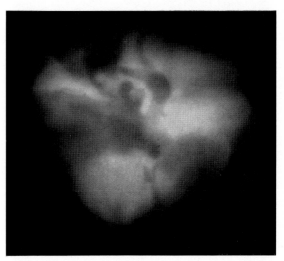

10.17   Tomograph corresponding to Fig. 10.16.

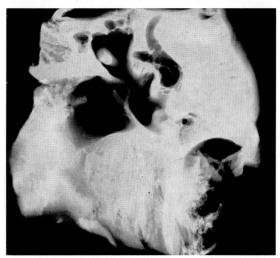

10.18   Microradiograph of semiaxial macrosection seen in Fig. 10.14 and 10.16.

Otosclerosis, Post-Stapedectomy

Figure 10.19 is a coronal tomograph at the level of the oval window of the same right temporal bone with otosclerosis as in Fig. 10.1–10.18. The thin line of the me-tallic prosthesis extends from the long process of the incus to the oval window.

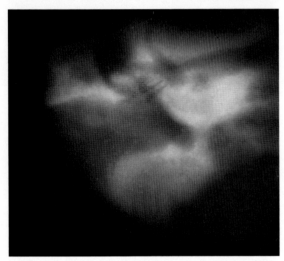

10.19   Coronal tomograph.

Histopathology

Figure 10.20 is a low-power photomicrograph of the section in Fig. 10.2 and 10.4.

Anterior to the oval window, there is an otosclerotic focus in the labyrinthine capsule between the facial nerve and the scala vestibuli of the basal coil of the cochlea. Figure 10.21 is a low-power photomicrograph of the section in Fig. 10.14 and 10.16.

This section lies at the posterior portion of the oval window. The posterior portion of the footplate is thickened by otosclerotic bone. There is an otosclerotic focus in the promontory which extends from the inferior margin of the oval window towards the round window niche.

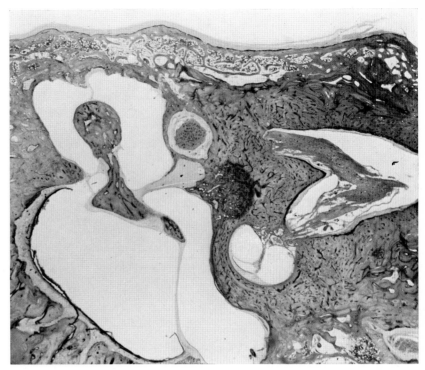

10.20   Photomicrograph of Fig. 10.2 and 10.4.

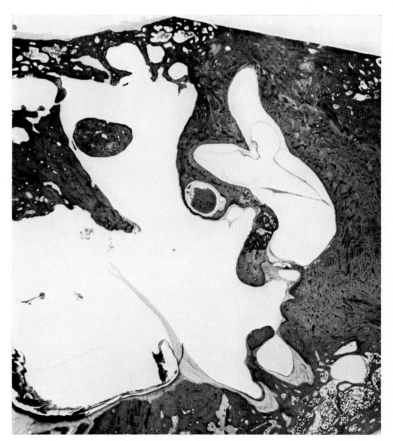

10.21   Photomicrograph of Fig. 10.14 and 10.16.

Chapter 11   Pathological Conditions Involving the Internal Auditory Canal

The tomographic study of the internal auditory canal is performed with sections two mm apart in the coronal and sagittal planes. The coronal sections are most satisfactory for the evaluation of the shape and vertical diameter of the canal, the length of the posterior canal wall, and status of the crista falciformis. The sagittal sections add details of utmost importance concerning the anteroposterior diameter of the canal and the condition of the cortex and porus of the canal.

The canals on both sides should be examined for comparison. When the two internal auditory canals of the same individual are compared, there is normally only a very slight difference in the measurements of the size and shape of the canals. However, there may be a great variation in measurements when the two canals of one normal individual are compared with the canals of another normal individual.

The normal diameter of the internal auditory canal ranges between 2 to 10 mm with a mean of 5.0 mm. A difference of 1 to 2 mm of any portion of one internal auditory canal in comparison to the corresponding segment of the canal of the opposite side is compatible with a variation of normal. An enlargement of 2 mm or more in the measurement of one canal compared with the opposite canal usually indicates a space occupying lesion on the enlarged side.

There are other important structures that must be considered in the evaluation of the internal auditory canal:

1) The posterior canal wall. This wall may become eroded and shortened by a tumor;

2) The outline of the canal which normally appears as a white cortical line surrounding the lumen of the canal. This white line may be disrupted by a pathological process;

3) The crista falciformis which divides the canal in two compartments. Normally the crista is located at or above the midpoint of the vertical diameter of the canal. A reversal of this ratio or an asymmetry by at least 2 mm in the position of the crista, when compared with the position of the crista on the normal side, is strongly suggestive of an intracanalicular mass.

One case is presented which shows an exostosis of the petrous pyramid adjacent to the internal auditory canal.

Exostosis of Posterior Surface of Temporal Bone

These illustrations show an exostosis of the posterior surface of a right, adult petrous bone at the level of the internal auditory canal. The sections lie in the sagittal plane and each section is 2 mm thick. Only the photographs and tomographs of the lateral surfaces of the two sections are shown.

The first 2 mm thick sagittal section lies at the level of the internal auditory canal, cochlea, carotid artery, eustachian tube and jugular fossa (Fig. 11.1–11.4).

A small broad-based exostosis protrudes from the posterior surface of the petrous pyramid opposite the lumen of the internal auditory canal.

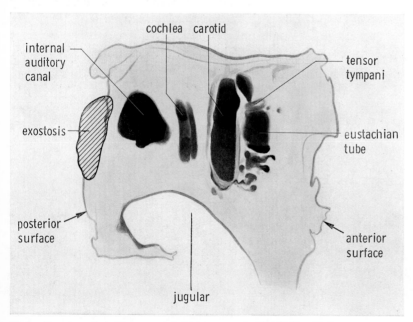

11.1   Drawing of structures and pathology seen in Fig. 11.2 to 11.4.

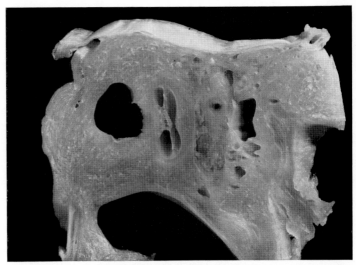

11.2   Photograph of lateral surface of a sagittal macrosection at the level of the internal auditory canal and the cochlea.

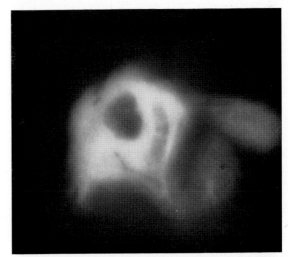

11.3   Tomograph corresponding to Fig. 11.2.

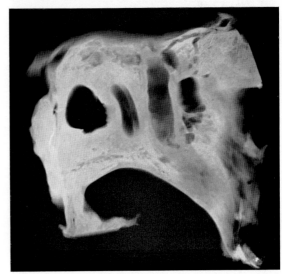

11.4   Microradiograph of the sagittal macrosection seen in Fig. 11.2.

Exostosis of Posterior Surface of Temporal Bone

Figures 11.5–11.8 show the exostosis in a 2 mm thick sagittal section of the same adult right temporal bone immediately medial to Fig. 11.1–11.4.

The section shows a medial extension on the posterior wall of the internal auditory canal of the exostosis appearing in Fig. 11.1–11.4.

The bony mass of the exostosis does not impinge on the lumen of the internal auditory canal.

These two consecutive coronal tomographs (Fig. 11.9 to 11.10), 1 mm apart are from the same temporal bone with an exostosis on the posterior surface in Fig. 11.1 to 11.8.

Figure 11.9 lies at the level of the posterior wall of the internal auditory canal, posterior portion of the vestibule and cochlear aqueduct.

The base of the exostosis appears above the internal auditory canal.

Figure 11.10, 1 mm posterior to Fig. 11.9, shows the entire exostosis on the posterosuperior wall of the petrous pyramid.

The inferior portion of the loop of the posterior semicircular canal begins to appear at this level.

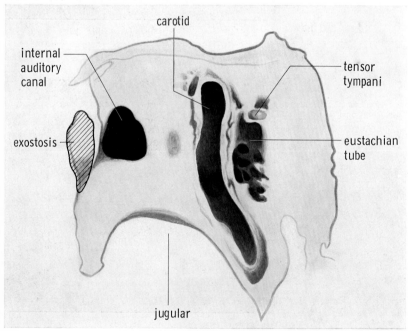

11.5   Drawing of structures and pathology seen in Fig. 11.6 to 11.8.

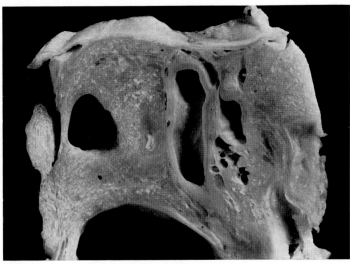

11.6   Photograph of latteral surface of the sagittal macrosection immediately medial to Fig. 11.2.

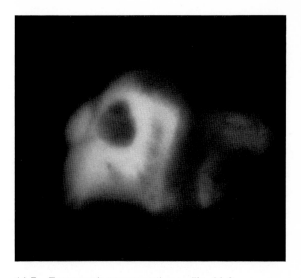

11.7   Tomograph corresponding to Fig. 11.6.

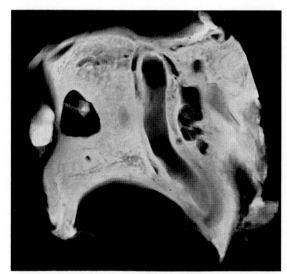

11.8   Microradiograph of the sagittal macrosection seen
in Fig. 11.6.

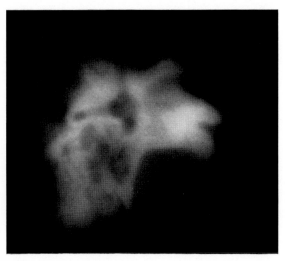

11.9   Coronal tomograph.

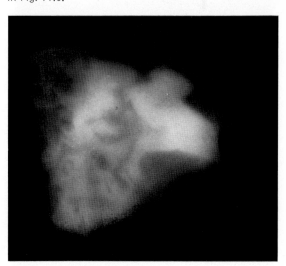

11.10   Coronal tomograph.

Index